BALANCE EXERCISES FOR SENIORS - MADE SIMPLE

SAFE, AT-HOME WORKOUTS TO IMPROVE BALANCE, STABILITY & PREVENT FALLS—EVEN IF YOU'VE NEVER EXERCISED BEFORE

LAUREL HARRIS

CONTENTS

INTRODUCTION

Three years ago, John, a spry 72-year-old with a love for gardening, found himself increasingly gripped by the fear of a simple misstep that could lead to a fall—a fear that started to eclipse his daily joys. Determined to reclaim his confidence and independence, John turned to a series of balance exercises. Within weeks, his stability improved, and he was also back in his garden, moving amongst his plants with a renewed sense of freedom. His story isn't just inspiring; it embodies the transformative journey that I've laid out in this book.

My personal journey into the world of balance for seniors began with my own grandmother. Watching her struggle with mobility and the anxiety of falling opened my eyes to the challenges that many seniors face daily. This experience ignited my passion to develop practical solutions that could make a real difference. It led me to years of research and collaboration with geriatric health and fitness experts, culminating in the program I am thrilled to share with you.

This book is designed to be your guide to regaining and maintaining balance through a 21-day program of simple, effective exercises. Each activity is crafted to fit into your daily routine, requiring just a few minutes but promising significant benefits. These are not just any exercises; they are backed by the latest scientific research and are tailored to address the unique needs of seniors. Whether you are looking to reduce your risk of falls, enhance your mobility, or simply improve your overall independence, this program is for you.

What sets this guide apart is its focus on accessibility and personalisation. Understanding that each individual's health and mobility levels vary, I've included modifications for each exercise to cater to a wide range of physical capabilities. This book also goes beyond physical exercises, offering advice on nutrition and mental health to support your overall well-being.

As you turn these pages, you'll find detailed, easy-to-follow instructions accompanied by illustrations that visually guide you through each exercise, ensuring you perform them safely and effectively. The layout of the book follows a logical progression, building your confidence as you advance through the weeks.

Let this be the moment you take control of your balance and, by extension, your life. I invite you to join me on this 21-day journey, not just to improve your balance but to embrace a fuller, more active future. Remember, it's never too late to start, and with just a few minutes a day, you can see profound changes in your stability and your confidence.

So, take this first step with me. Together, let's move towards a life marked not by fear and restriction, but by stability and freedom. Welcome to your new path to independence through balance.

CHAPTER 1

UNDERSTANDING BALANCE AND AGING

D ID YOU KNOW THAT one in four Americans aged 65 and over falls each year? While this statistic might seem a bit daunting, there's good news: many falls are preventable. And that's precisely what we're here to talk about—understanding the intricate dance of balance that your body performs every day and how you can fine-tune it as you age. This chapter is designed to peel back the layers of how balance works, why it often declines as we age, and most importantly, how specific exercises can significantly improve your balance and reduce the risk of falls. By understanding the science behind balance, you're better equipped to take proactive steps towards maintaining it.

1.1 The Science of Balance in Seniors

Balance Mechanics Explained

Balance isn't just about not falling over; it's a complex mechanism involving several systems in your body. The primary players in maintaining balance are your vestibular system (located in your inner ear), your vision, and proprioception, which is your body's ability to sense its position in space. Together, these systems send constant signals to your brain about your body's position relative to the world around you. For instance, the vestibular system informs your brain about movements and changes in the position of your head, while your eyes help you navigate the space around you, and proprioceptors in your muscles and skin send information about your limbs' positions. This intricate network works seamlessly to keep you upright and stable.

However, as we age, these systems can start to show signs of wear and tear. The fluid in your inner ear that helps monitor the motion may diminish, proprioceptors might become less sensitive, and vision can deteriorate. When these changes occur, the brain gets less accurate information, making it harder to maintain balance. This is why the risk of falling increases as we age, and it underscores the critical importance of targeted exercises that can help mitigate these effects.

Age-related Deterioration

As mentioned, the decline in the efficiency of balance-related systems is a natural part of aging. However, it doesn't mean that falling is inevitable. Understanding this deterioration is the first step in combating it. For example, reduced fluid in the inner ear affects your vestibular system's ability to accurately detect movement and can lead to vertigo or dizziness. Similarly, less sensitive proprioceptors might not alert you quickly enough if you're starting to tip over, delaying your reaction time to catch yourself.

Impact of Exercise on Neuroplasticity

Here's where the real magic happens: exercise can significantly improve your balance, thanks to something called neuroplasticity. This is your brain's ability to reorganise itself by forming new neural connections throughout life. Balance exercises stimulate these connections, particularly in the parts of your brain involved in motion and spatial orientation. Regular balance training can help sharpen your reflexes, improve your muscle strength, and ultimately, enhance your body's ability to control its position. This is particularly crucial for seniors, as enhanced neuroplasticity through targeted exercises can lead to substantial improvements in overall stability and mobility.

Research and Case Studies

The effectiveness of balance training isn't just anecdotal; it's backed by science. Numerous studies have shown that balance exercise programs for seniors can lead to improvements in stability, a reduction in the number of falls, and enhancements in the quality of life. For instance, a study published in the Journal of Geriatric Physical Therapy found that seniors who engaged in balance training saw a significant improvement in their ability to perform daily activities and reported fewer falls. Moreover, these exercises not only improve physical balance but also contribute to enhanced confidence in performing everyday activities, thus reducing the fear of falling.

Incorporating balance exercises into your daily routine doesn't require gym equipment or vast spaces; many exercises can be performed in the comfort of your living room. By understanding the underlying science of balance and actively engaging in exercises aimed at improving it, you empower yourself to lead a safer and more active life as you age. And remember, it's never too late to start. Whether you're looking to enhance your current fitness routine or you're starting from scratch, the key is consistency and the willingness to stick with it. Every bit of movement counts towards building a steadier, more confident you.

1.2 Common Age-Related Changes in Mobility

As we age, our bodies undergo several changes that can impact our mobility. This isn't just about moving slower; it's about how the structural and functional shifts in our muscles, joints, and bones can affect our ability to move and balance as we once did. Muscle strength declines, often due to reduced physical activity and changes in muscle composition. Joint flexibility decreases as the cartilage that helps joints move smoothly wears down over time, and our bones lose density, which can make them more fragile. These physical changes can make it challenging to perform everyday activities that were once taken for granted.

Imagine a simple activity like climbing stairs. For a young person, this is a straightforward task, but as you age, reduced muscle strength and joint stiffness can turn this everyday activity into a challenge. Walking on an uneven path can become a perilous journey because the body's decreased ability to quickly respond to changes in terrain can increase the risk of falls. These examples highlight how age-related changes in mobility can directly impact daily life, making activities that require balance, strength, and coordination more difficult.

However, it's not all doom and gloom. Engaging in regular balance and strength exercises can significantly slow down or even counteract these declines in mobility. Exercise is like a tonic for your muscles and joints. It keeps them conditioned and the nerves that control them sharp, ensuring that movements remain more fluid and less prone to injury. Strength training can help rebuild muscle mass and increase bone density, reducing the risk of osteoporosis. Flexibility exercises keep joints limber, decreasing the likelihood of pain and stiffness.

Personalising these exercises is crucial because everyone ages differently. What works for one person might not work for another. Tailoring exercises to individual mobility levels and health conditions ensures that each person can participate safely and effectively in maintaining their mobility. For instance, someone with mild joint pain might benefit from low-impact activities such as swimming or cycling, which provide resistance without putting too much strain on the joints. Meanwhile, someone else might require targeted strength training to help rebuild muscle lost due to prolonged inactivity.

Incorporating these exercises into your routine doesn't have to be a chore. Many can be seamlessly integrated into daily activities. For example, while waiting for the kettle to boil, you can perform calf raises or stand on one leg to practice balance. Every little bit helps, and the key is consistency. Regularly engaging in these activities can make a noticeable difference in how you navigate daily tasks, providing not only physical benefits but also boosting your confidence and independence as you age.

Regular participation in balance and strength activities is more than just a preventative measure; it's a way to ensure that your later years are as active and enjoyable as the earlier ones. It's about maintaining the freedom to move comfortably and safely through your world, which is essential for physical health and emotional well-being. So, while the body may naturally face challenges as it ages, there are effective strategies to manage these changes and maintain a vibrant, active lifestyle. Each step taken to improve your balance and mobility is a step towards preserving your independence and quality of life.

1.3 Psychological Impacts of Falling Fears

The fear of falling, often referred to as 'fear of falling syndrome,' is not just about the physical act of a fall; it encompasses a pervasive dread that can significantly limit your life's quality and scope. This fear is remarkably common among seniors, where even those who have never fallen might begin to worry excessively about the possibility. The concern isn't unfounded, as falls are a leading cause of injury among older adults. However, the fear itself can initiate a limiting cycle: you might start avoiding activities you think could lead to a fall, such as walking, shopping, or socialising. This reduction in activity leads to physical de-conditioning, which ironically increases the risk of falling. It's a self-fulfilling prophecy: the fear of falling can bring about the circumstances that make a fall more likely.

This cycle can have profound psychological consequences. The constant worry about a potential fall can lead to anxiety, which in itself can be debilitating. Anxiety might cause you to be overly cautious and tense, which can interfere with your balance and make you even more prone to accidents. Moreover, the social withdrawal that often accompanies this fear can lead to isolation and loneliness, which are significant risk factors for mental health issues such as depression. Imagine missing out on your grandchild's birthday party or a coffee date with old friends because the fear of stepping out feels overwhelming. These missed opportunities for joy can profoundly impact your overall well-being and happiness.

However, there is a beacon of hope in this scenario: exercise, specifically balance exercises. Engaging regularly in balance-focused activities can significantly mitigate this fear by enhancing your physical stability. When you feel more stable, you're less likely to fall, and just as importantly, you're less likely to fear falling. Each small success in these exercises can build your confidence, slowly breaking down the mental barriers erected by fear. Picture this: each time you successfully complete a balance exercise, it's another brick removed from the wall of fear, gradually letting the light of confidence back into your life. Through consistent practice, these exercises empower you, giving back the control that fear has taken away.

Supportive environments play a crucial role in this transformation. Encouragement from friends, family, and community groups can be tremendously motivating. Participating in group exercises, whether at a local community centre or even a simple walking group in the neighbourhood, provides not only physical benefits but also social interaction, which can alleviate feelings of isolation. Knowing you have a network of support, and people who understand and encourage your efforts to overcome your fears can make all the difference. They can offer encouragement on tough days and celebrate your successes, making the journey less daunting. In many cases, they can also provide practical support, like accompanying you on walks until you feel confident enough to do them alone, ensuring safety while also fostering independence.

By understanding the psychological impacts of the fear of falling and actively engaging in strategies to combat it, you can maintain not only your physical health but also your independence and quality of life. This approach isn't just about preventing falls; it's about breaking the cycle of fear and reclaiming the joy and freedom in your daily activities. With each step you take on this path, remember that it's not just about avoiding falls—it's about rising to the full height of your potential, no matter your age.

1.4 The Benefits of Maintaining an Active Lifestyle

Have you ever noticed how a day spent moving and doing leaves you feeling better, not just physically but mentally too? It's not just about burning calories or strengthening muscles; leading an active lifestyle works wonders across multiple facets of your life, especially as we age. Engaging regularly in physical activities can boost cardiovascular health, enhance muscular strength, and fortify your bones, all of which are integral to maintaining a good balance.

When you keep your body moving, you're essentially ensuring that your heart stays robust, pumping efficiently and improving blood circulation. This is crucial because good circulation contributes to the overall vitality of all bodily functions and plays a significant role in maintaining muscle strength and health. Stronger muscles support your joints and bones better, reducing the wear and tear that comes with age. Moreover, activities like walking, swimming, or even gardening can help increase bone density. This is particularly important to combat conditions like osteoporosis, which seniors are prone to due to the natural decrease in bone mass with age. Each step you take, each lap you swim, isn't just exercise; it's an investment in your body's bank of health, ensuring you remain agile and less prone to falls.

Now, let's chat about the brain benefits, shall we? Staying active isn't just a boon for the body but also for the mind. Engaging in regular physical activity has been shown to sharpen memory, boost attention, and enhance problem-solving skills. This is because exercise helps to increase blood flow to the brain, which in turn aids in the growth of new brain cells and the connections between them. This can be particularly noticeable in senior years, where cognitive functions might naturally decline. By incorporating activities like puzzles during a walk or strategy games on the move, you're not only giving your body a workout but also challenging your brain, keeping it as fit as your physique.

But perhaps one of the most overlooked aspects of an active lifestyle is its impact on emotional and social well-being. Feelings of loneliness and isolation can sometimes creep up as we age, but staying active provides a powerful antidote. Group activities, whether it's a dance class, a weekly walking group, or a yoga session at the local community centre, offer wonderful opportunities to interact with others, share experiences, and build friendships. The emotional boost from such interactions is invaluable; it uplifts spirits and can even alleviate symptoms of depression and anxiety. Moreover, the sense of community and belonging that comes from social interactions helps reinforce the support network that is crucial in later years, providing both emotional security and practical assistance when needed.

Connecting these dots, it becomes clear that the independence treasured in later years is greatly supported by an active lifestyle. Regular exercise doesn't just keep the body strong; it keeps the spirit resilient and self-reliant. The ability to move around, engage in activities, and interact with others without feeling hindered by physical limitations is a cornerstone of quality life as we age. It allows seniors to enjoy a sense of freedom and control over their lives, continue to contribute to their communities, and enjoy new experiences without the shadow of helplessness that often looms with age-related physical decline.

So, think of an active lifestyle as a multifaceted tool in your kit for aging well. It's about dancing to your favourite songs, taking brisk evening walks, playing with your grandchildren, and so much more. Each active moment enhances your physical, mental, and emotional health, weaving together a tapestry of a well-lived senior life that's full of joy, health, and independence.

1.5 Assessing Your Current Balance Ability

When it comes to maintaining your balance, knowing where you stand—quite literally—can be your first step towards improvement. It's essential to assess your balance capabilities periodically, which helps in tailoring your exercises effectively and monitoring progress. Think of it as a personal baseline from which you can measure every small success along the way.

Let's start with some simple methods you can use at home to assess your balance. A popular and effective test is the 'single-leg stand.'

Here's how you do it: stand behind a sturdy chair and hold onto the back of it. Lift one foot off the ground and try to balance on the other foot. Count how long you can hold the position without grabbing the chair for support. Try this on both legs. It's a quick and simple way to gauge your balance and track improvements over time.

Another method is the 'walk-and-turn' test, where you walk in a straight line, then turn and walk back. This test is not only about balance but also tests your ability to coordinate and control your movements.

Understanding the importance of regular check-ins on your balance is crucial. Think of these as routine maintenance for your body, much like you'd service a car. As you progress through the exercises in this book, these assessments help you see tangible proof of your improvement. They can also alert you to any declines in balance, prompting you to adjust your exercise plan or seek further advice. Regular balance checks keep you motivated and on track, providing a personal record of just how far you have come. They're also incredibly encouraging, turning abstract concepts of 'improvement' into something you can see and feel.

In today's tech-savvy world, several tools and apps can help you monitor your balance and mobility. These range from simple apps that use your smartphone's motion sensors to more sophisticated balance boards that connect to your phone via Bluetooth. These tools provide a more detailed analysis of your balance, offering insights into areas like weight distribution and postural sway. While not essential, they can be a fun and useful way to get more data about your physical state.

However, nothing beats the personalised guidance that a professional can offer. Consulting with healthcare providers or physical therapists is highly advisable, especially if you're experiencing significant balance issues. These professionals can perform comprehensive assessments using equipment and techniques that are more sophisticated than what we can do at home. They can also provide you with a personalized exercise plan tailored to your specific needs. This is particularly important if you have a medical condition affecting your balance, such as vertigo or a recent surgery.

Remember, these assessments are not just about preventing falls; they're about enhancing your overall mobility and quality of life. They give you the confidence to participate in the activities you love, secure in the knowledge that you're building a stronger, more stable foundation. Whether you're perfecting your garden, playing with your grandchildren, or simply navigating the grocery store, every step you take with improved balance is a step toward a fuller, more active life. So, take these initial assessments seriously and make them a regular part of your routine. They're your first step on the path to a steadier, more confident you. I will see you in the next chapter where we will go through **Preparing for Balance Training.**

Chapter 2

Preparing For Balance Training

I MAGINE SETTING UP A little sanctuary where every corner is designed to encourage your balance and mobility goals. This isn't just any ordinary space; it's where you'll reclaim strength and confidence, and perhaps even carve out a few moments of joy in your daily routine. Just as a painter needs a well-organized studio to create art, you need a safe, comfortable space to work on your masterpiece—your mobility and independence.

2.1 Safety First: Setting Up Your Exercise Space

Choosing the Right Location

Finding the right spot for your exercises is the first step in creating a safe exercise environment. You'll want to select a space that is not only spacious enough for you to move freely without bumping into furniture but also one that has a non-slip floor to prevent any unwanted slides or falls. For many, a living room or a cleared-out section of a family room works perfectly. It's important that this area is free of clutter like loose rugs, electrical cords, or any small objects that could become tripping hazards. A good tip is to have enough room to stretch your arms out fully in all directions—imagine being at the centre of a bubble that extends out from your fingertips.

Safety Modifications

Once you've picked your spot, it's time to make a few quick safety tweaks. First, please make sure to secure any rugs with double-sided tape or slip-resistant backing to keep them firmly in place. Good lighting is crucial, so ensure that the space is well-lit to avoid any shadows or dark corners where you could misstep. If you're using equipment like a chair for exercises, make sure it's sturdy and won't slide on your floor. Sometimes, placing a bit of rubber matting under chair legs can add that extra grip and stability you need.

Creating a Safe Fall Zone

Even with the best precautions, slips or stumbles can happen, and that's perfectly okay. To prepare for this, consider setting up a 'safe fall zone' by arranging soft mats or thick cushions around your exercise area. This is particularly important if you're at a higher risk of falling or if you're trying out new exercises that challenge your balance significantly. Think of this zone as a little buffer area—it's there to catch you if you stumble, making any falls as soft as possible.

Emergency Preparedness

Lastly, let's talk about preparedness. Always have a phone accessible in your exercise space. You might never need it, but it should be there, just in case. Program it with emergency contacts, including family members, close friends, or your doctor's office. This way, help is just a call away if you ever need it. Additionally, consider wearing a medical alert device if you're often alone at home; these can be invaluable in alerting emergency services if you fall and can't get to a phone.

Creating this safe exercise space might take a little bit of time and effort, but it's absolutely worth it. Think of it as setting the stage for success. Here, in your personalised zone, you're free to focus purely on your exercises, secure in the knowledge that you've minimised risks and maximised safety. This peace of mind is crucial, not just for your physical safety but for your confidence too. It's much easier to commit to your balance exercises when you know you've done everything possible to create a safe environment. So take a little time to set up your space.

Once it's done, you'll have a dedicated spot that invites you to work on your balance every day, safely and effectively.

2.2 Essential Equipment for Balance Exercises at Home

As you embark on this rewarding path to enhance your balance, having the right equipment by your side can make all the difference. It's like having the best tools in a toolkit; they don't just make the job easier but also more effective. Let's start with the basics—the must-haves for anyone beginning balance exercises at home. First, a sturdy chair is invaluable. It serves not just for seated exercises but also as a stable support for various standing exercises. Opt for one without wheels and with a solid backrest for maximum safety. Next, consider a non-slip yoga mat. This isn't just for yoga; its grip and cushioning make it perfect for a range of exercises, providing you with a safe, defined space that supports your movements. And let's not forget about footwear. Comfortable, supportive shoes are crucial. They should have a good grip and offer proper support to your arches, helping you maintain balance while protecting your feet during exercises.

Now, if you're ready to take things up a notch, there are some more advanced tools that can really enhance your training. Balance pads, for instance, add an extra level of challenge to your workouts. These thick foam mats increase the difficulty of your balance exercises by creating an unstable surface, forcing your muscles to work harder to stabilise your body. It's fantastic for advanced balance training and can significantly improve your proprioception—that's your body's ability to sense its position in space. Foam rollers, on the other hand, are great not just for balance but also for muscle relaxation and improving flexibility. They can be used in a variety of ways, from stability exercises to deep-tissue massages to soothe sore muscles. Then there are stability balls. These large, inflatable balls are terrific for engaging multiple muscle groups. Exercises on a stability ball require you to maintain balance, which activates and strengthens the core muscles—key players in good balance.

For those of you who are mindful of budget or simply prefer a do-it-yourself approach, there are plenty of cost-effective alternatives that don't skimp on effectiveness. Instead of a yoga mat, a large towel or a blanket could provide a temporary solution. It might not offer the same grip or padding but can work for someone just starting out or as a makeshift option when travelling. For weights, look no further than your kitchen—water bottles or canned goods can serve as excellent substitutes for hand weights. They're great for adding a little resistance to your exercises, helping build strength and stability.

Storing and maintaining your equipment is just as important as using it. Proper storage not only keeps your space tidy and safe but also extends the life of your equipment. Keep your mats rolled up and out of the way when not in use, and store any small equipment like weights or foam rollers in a basket or box. Regularly check your items for any signs of wear and tear, especially on items like stability balls or balance pads that could pose a safety risk if damaged. Cleaning your equipment is also key, particularly for items you use frequently. A simple wipe-down with a disinfectant can help keep everything hygienic and in top condition.

By equipping yourself with the right tools and taking care of them, you enhance your ability to perform each balance exercise safely and effectively. This preparation not only sets you up for success in your balance training but also ensures that you can continue these practices safely as part of your lifestyle, keeping you active and agile in the comfort of your home.

2.3 Warm-Ups and Cool-Downs: Protecting Your Muscles and Joints

Think of your body as a car in the chilly early morning hours. You wouldn't just start it and zoom off; instead, you'd let it idle for a bit, allowing the engine to warm up for a smoother, safer ride. This is much like your muscles and joints when it comes to exercise. Starting your balance routine without a proper warm-up is akin to that cold start—it might work, but it increases the risk of strains or injuries. Warm-ups gently prepare your body for the activity ahead, making the muscles more pliable and responsive, which not only enhances your performance but also shields you from potential harm.

A good warm-up gradually revs up your cardiovascular system by raising your body temperature and increasing blood flow to your muscles. Consider simple, gentle stretching and mobility exercises that don't demand too much from your body right out of the gate. For instance, you might start with some shoulder rolls or arm circles, which open up the upper body, followed by marching in place to get the blood flowing to your legs. These activities gently coax your body into exercise mode, preparing both your muscles and your mind for the balance exercises to follow. It's about giving your body a heads-up that you're about to ask more of it, ensuring everything is nicely tuned and ready to perform.

Now, transitioning into specific warm-up exercises tailored for seniors, focus on movements that are gentle yet effective in preparing you for balance training. A great exercise to include is the toe tap. Standing behind your sturdy chair for support, slowly tap your toes on the ground in front of you, alternating feet. This not only warms up the lower leg muscles but also engages your sense of balance in a controlled manner. Another excellent warm-up is the side leg raise. Holding onto your chair for support, gently lift one leg out to the side and back down, repeating several times before switching to the other leg. This exercise activates the hip and outer thigh areas, which are crucial for maintaining balance.

Moving on, let's talk about the importance of cooling down, which is just as crucial as warming up. After engaging in balance exercises, your body needs a moment to regroup and shift back to its normal state. Cooling down allows your heart rate to return to its resting pace gradually and helps prevent muscle stiffness and soreness, which can be a deterrent to continuing with an exercise routine. This gradual wind-down period is your body's chance to recover and reset, which is especially important after putting it through the paces of balance training.

For an effective cool-down, focus on exercises and stretches that relax and lengthen the muscles you've just worked. A simple yet effective cool-down stretch is the calf stretch. Place your hands on the wall or the back of your sturdy chair, step one foot back, and gently press your heel to the floor until you feel a stretch in the back of your leg. Hold this for a few breaths, then switch legs. Another beneficial cool-down is the seated forward bend. Sitting on a chair, slowly lean forward, letting your hands slide toward your feet, and hold this position to stretch your lower back and hamstrings gently.

These cooldown routines not only aid in physical recovery but also provide a moment to reflect on the workout you've completed, fostering a sense of accomplishment and encouraging you to maintain this beneficial practice. Incorporating these stretches and relaxation techniques ensures that your transition back to your daily activities is as smooth and comfortable as possible, keeping your muscles flexible and responsive for your next balance session. By dedicating time to proper warm-ups and cool-downs, you're not just performing exercises; you're investing in your body's long-term health and mobility, ensuring it serves you well for all your daily adventures.

2.4 Understanding and Managing Chronic Pain During Exercises

When it comes to staying active, managing pain is a crucial aspect, especially for seniors who might already be dealing with chronic conditions. It's about knowing your body and understanding the messages it sends you. Pain during exercise can be a normal part of increasing physical activity, especially if your muscles aren't used to it. However, not all pain is created equal, and distinguishing between 'good' pain, which is normal discomfort from exertion, and 'bad' pain, which could signal an injury or an underlying issue, is key to exercising safely.

'Good' pain might feel like a mild burn or fatigue in your muscles during or immediately after a workout and generally subsides fairly quickly with rest. This type of pain is a natural response to your muscles getting stronger. On the other hand, 'bad' pain is sharp, stabbing, or persistent discomfort that continues or worsens with activity. This type of pain might indicate something more serious, like a strain or joint issue, and should not be ignored. It's crucial to listen to your body and recognise when pain changes from being a typical workout burn to a warning signal.

Adjusting your exercises to manage pain effectively is crucial and entirely achievable. For instance, if a particular movement causes discomfort, modifying it can often allow you to continue exercising without pain. Let's say a standing balance exercise is causing knee pain; switching to a seated version can often alleviate stress on your knees while still strengthening your core and improving your balance. Using props like chairs for support during standing exercises can also reduce the load on painful joints or muscles. The key here is to adapt exercises to meet your body where it is, not where you think it should be. This customisation ensures that you continue to benefit from activity without putting yourself at risk of injury.

In terms of non-exercise-related techniques for managing pain, several strategies can be effective. Proper hydration is crucial; sometimes, muscle cramps and pains are related to dehydration. Ensuring you drink enough water throughout the day can help keep your tissues healthy and elastic, which can prevent pain. Adequate sleep is another pillar of pain management. During sleep, your body repairs itself which includes recovery from the microtears in muscle fibers that occur during exercise. Ensuring you get a restorative night's sleep can enhance this natural recovery process and reduce pain. Sometimes, despite these measures, pain might persist, indicating it's time to consult with healthcare professionals. They can offer tailored advice, possibly including physical therapy or appropriate medications, to help manage your pain effectively.

Knowing when to stop is perhaps the most crucial strategy in your pain management toolkit. If you experience sharp or severe pain during exercise, or if mild pain doesn't improve with rest and modifications, it's essential to stop and seek professional advice. Continuing to exercise through severe pain is not only counterproductive but can also lead to more severe injuries. Remember, the goal of incorporating balance and exercise into your daily routine is to enhance your quality of life, not to push through pain to the point of injury. Your body is your most valuable asset, and treating it with care and respect by heeding pain signals is paramount.

Navigating the complexities of pain during exercise isn't just about making physical adjustments; it's about fostering a deeper connection with your body. It involves listening intently to its signals and responding with kindness, whether through modifying your exercise routine, incorporating supportive strategies like hydration and sleep, or seeking professional help when needed. This approach ensures that you can continue to enjoy the benefits of an active lifestyle, which includes maintaining your independence and vitality, without being sidelined by pain. Remember, every step taken to manage pain is a step towards maintaining your overall health and well-being.

2.5 Tailoring Exercises to Your Health Conditions

When it comes to balance exercises, one size does not fit all, especially when you are contending with health conditions that could affect your mobility or safety. Conditions such as arthritis, osteoporosis, or cardiovascular issues each come with their own set of challenges and precautions, making it crucial to tailor your exercise routine to fit your personal health landscape. For instance, if arthritis is part of your daily life, high-impact activities might exacerbate pain or inflammation. Instead, you could focus on low-impact balance exercises that improve stability without stressing your joints.

Osteoporosis requires a careful approach to physical activity to enhance bone density while avoiding fractures. Weight-bearing exercises, which force you to work against gravity, can be beneficial in strengthening bones and improving balance. However, these need to be performed with a focus on safety to prevent falls. On the other hand, if you're managing cardiovascular issues, exercises that elevate your heart rate should be approached with caution. Balancing exercises that can be performed seated or with the support of a chair are excellent as they reduce the risk of sudden drops in blood pressure, which can lead to dizziness or falls.

The key to successfully integrating balance exercises into your routine, considering these conditions, is regular consultation with healthcare professionals. A physical therapist or your doctor can help create a personalised exercise plan that not only respects but embraces your body's current state, optimising your efforts and ensuring safety. They can offer modifications that tailor exercises to your needs, suggest the best types of activities based on your health, and provide guidance on how to progress safely.

Monitoring changes in your health status is another critical aspect. As we age, our bodies continue to change, and an exercise program that works for you now might need adjustments down the line. Regular check-ups and open communication with your healthcare provider can help you stay on top of these changes and modify your exercise regimen accordingly. This proactive approach ensures that your balance exercises continue to benefit you without causing harm.

Integrating therapeutic exercises into your routine can also play a significant role in managing specific conditions. For example, Tai Chi has been shown to improve balance and stability in those with Parkinson's Disease and similar neurological conditions. Its gentle, flowing movements improve muscle strength, flexibility, and reflexes, all of which contribute to better balance. For those dealing with arthritis, water aerobics can be a wonderful way to improve balance and strength. The buoyancy of the water reduces stress on the joints while providing resistance, making it an ideal setting for gentle balance training.

By personalising your exercise routine to fit your unique health needs, not only do you enhance your safety and effectiveness, but you also ensure that your path to improved balance is as enjoyable and beneficial as possible. This personalized approach empowers you to maintain your independence and keep engaging actively in life, knowing that your exercise routine supports your health in the best possible way.

And there you have it—the groundwork for safe and effective balance training tailored just for you. Remember, every step you take in preparation is a step toward a more balanced and fulfilling life. Next up, we'll dive into the fun stuff: beginning your balance exercises! Stay tuned as we guide you through simple yet effective movements designed to set you firmly on your feet.

CHAPTER 3

BEGINNER BALANCE EXERCISES

WELCOME TO THE EXCITING start of your hands-on journey towards improved balance and stability! This chapter is all about easing into balance exercises that are not only simple and safe but also incredibly effective. Imagine each exercise as a stepping stone towards a more confident and independent you. We're going to start this adventure with some beginner-friendly exercises that you can do right from the comfort of your chair. These exercises are perfect if you're just getting started or if standing for long periods is a bit challenging. So, grab a sturdy chair, and let's gently ease into your balance training.

3.1 Seated Exercises to Enhance Stability

Chair-Based Leg Lifts

Seated leg lifts are a fantastic way to begin strengthening your lower body and core, which are crucial for good balance. Here's how to do them:

- Sit upright in your chair with your feet flat on the ground. Engage your abdominal muscles as you slowly lift one leg straight out in front of you.

- Keep the leg in the air for five to ten seconds before slowly lowering it back down.

- Repeat this three times, then switch to the other leg.

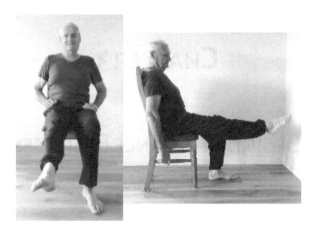

This exercise not only strengthens the muscles in your thighs and abdomen but also challenges your balance in a safe, controlled way. As you progress, you can increase the challenge by adding a light ankle weight, but always listen to your body and move to the next step only when you feel comfortable.

Arm Raises and Extensions

While your lower body is essential for balance, your upper body plays a vital role too. Strengthening your arms and shoulders can help you better control your movements and maintain stability.

- For this exercise, remain seated in your chair with your arms at your sides. Slowly lift your arms straight in front of you, up to shoulder height, hold for five to ten seconds, then gently lower them back down.

- Repeat this three times.

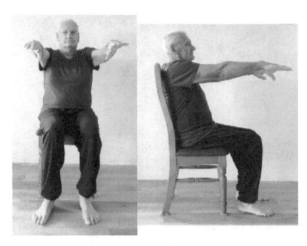

These movements help strengthen your shoulder and arm muscles, which are important for tasks like lifting groceries or even pushing yourself up from a chair. Plus, strong arms and shoulders can help you catch yourself if you start to fall, potentially reducing the risk of injury.

Seated Twists for Core Engagement

Your core muscles, which include your abdomen and lower back, are pivotal for maintaining balance. Let's engage them with some gentle seated twists.

- Sit up straight in your chair, feet flat on the floor, and place your hands behind your head or across your chest. Slowly twist your upper body to the right as far as is comfortable, hold for five to ten seconds, and then return to the centre. Follow the same instructions but on the left side.

- Repeat three times.

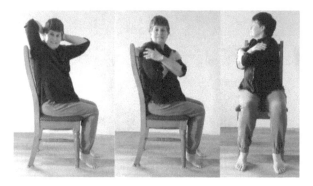

This twisting motion helps strengthen your core muscles, making it easier to maintain your balance during daily activities. It's also a great way to increase the flexibility and range of motion in your spine.

Breathing and Posture Alignment

One of the simplest yet most effective ways to enhance the effectiveness of your exercises is to focus on your breathing and posture. Proper posture aligns your body, promoting better balance, while deep breathing ensures your muscles get the oxygen they need to perform at their best.

- Here's what to do: sit up straight in your chair, shoulders back, and imagine a string pulling you up from the top of your head. As you perform each exercise, breathe deeply and steadily. Inhale slowly through your nose, and exhale through your mouth. This not only helps keep you relaxed but also engages your core and stabilizes your spine, enhancing the overall effectiveness of your exercises.

By incorporating these simple seated exercises into your routine, you're taking important steps towards improving your balance and stability. Each movement is designed to build the strength and coordination needed for everyday activities, reducing your risk of falls and boosting your confidence.

What's wonderful about these exercises is that they can be done anytime, whether you're watching TV, having a coffee, or taking a break from reading.

They're a great starting point for anyone looking to enhance their balance and a perfect foundation for more advanced exercises as you progress in your balance training. So, take it slow, be consistent, and remember, every little bit counts towards a more balanced you.

3.2 Simple Standing Stability Workouts

Let's shift the gear a bit and get you standing with some easy yet impactful exercises that focus on building your stability while you're up and about.

Starting with a classic but golden move, the wall push-up, this is an exercise that packs a lot of punch in terms of benefits.

Wall Push-ups

Wall push-ups are a fantastic way to strengthen your upper body without the strain of traditional floor push-ups, which can be tough on your wrists and shoulders.

- Here's how you do them: stand an arm's length in front of a wall with your feet shoulder-width apart.

- Place your palms flat against the wall at shoulder height and width. Bending your elbows, lean your body towards the wall, keeping your feet firmly on the ground.

- Push back to the starting position. As you press away from the wall, you engage not just your arms and chest but also your core, which plays a huge role in your overall balance.

- Repeat ten times.

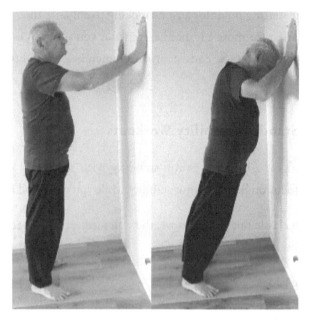

Strengthening these muscles helps you maintain better posture and stability, making everyday tasks feel easier and safer.

Standing heel-to-toe

Moving on to a balance-specific exercise, let's try the standing heel-to-toe pose. This exercise is perfect for improving your balance and body awareness, which are key to feeling confident in your movements.

- Begin by standing upright next to a stable chair or counter that you can use for support if needed.

- Place your right foot directly in front of your left foot so that the heel of your right foot touches the toe of your left foot. If this feels too challenging, start with your feet slightly apart, and gradually move them closer together as your confidence grows.

- Hold this position for as long as you can manage, then switch feet. This pose not only challenges your balance but also trains your body to manage instability, which is crucial in preventing falls.

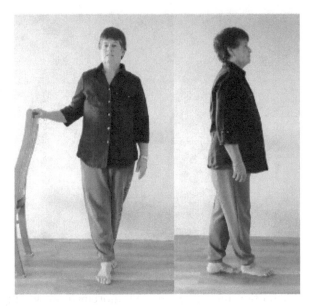

Side-to-side weight shifting

Let's add a dynamic element to your routine with some side-to-side weight shifting. This exercise is excellent for building ankle stability and improving your ability to control and correct your balance if you start to tip over.

- Stand with your feet hip-width apart, near a chair or countertop for support. Slowly shift your weight to your right foot, lifting your left foot off the ground just a bit. Hold for three to five seconds, then shift your weight to your left foot, lifting your right foot.

- Continue shifting your weight from side to side, gradually increasing the time you balance on one foot as you get more comfortable.

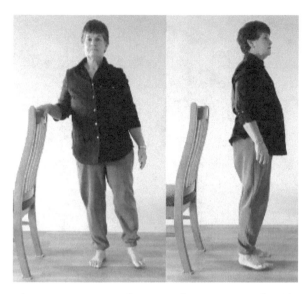

This side-to-side motion mimics the natural movement of walking, making it incredibly practical for everyday life.

Throughout these exercises, using a stable chair or counter for support is not just a safety measure but also a fantastic confidence booster. It's there if you need it, allowing you to focus on performing the exercises correctly without the fear of falling.

Over time, as your balance improves, you might find that you rely on that chair less and less, which is a wonderful sign of progress.

But remember, there's no rush. The goal is to build your balance safely and steadily, ensuring that each step forward is taken with confidence.

These standing stability workouts are designed to be accessible and effective, providing you with the tools you need to enhance your balance through simple, everyday movements.

Whether you're doing wall push-ups to strengthen your upper body, practising the heel-to-toe pose to better your balance, or shifting your weight from side to side to improve ankle stability, each exercise contributes significantly to your ability to stand strong and steady.

So take your time, enjoy the process, and celebrate each small victory along the way. Each effort you make is a building block in your foundation of stability and confidence, keeping you active and independent.

3.3 Gentle Tai Chi Movements for Beginners

Tai Chi, often described as meditation in motion, is not just exercise—it's a gentle way to fight stress and improve balance. This ancient Chinese tradition, originally developed for self-defence, has evolved into a graceful form of exercise that involves a series of movements performed in a slow, focused manner, accompanied by deep breathing.

Each posture flows into the next without pause, ensuring that your body is in constant motion. The philosophy behind Tai Chi is to foster a calm and tranquil mind, focusing on the flow of energy through your body, which practitioners call 'qi' or 'chi'. By integrating mind, body, and spirit, Tai Chi promotes not only physical balance but also mental health.

Starting with the basics, the hand movements in Tai Chi are simple yet profound. They require you to move with precision and harmony.

For beginners, especially seniors, you can perform these movements either standing or seated.

Cloud hands

- One basic movement is the "cloud hands" which involves passing your hands across your body in a gentle waving motion, as if softly pushing clouds across the sky.

- This not only aids in upper body coordination but also helps in focusing your mind, reducing stress levels.

- Do this motion for 30 seconds to one minute.

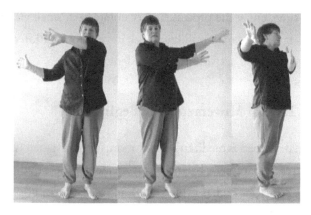

The beauty of these movements lies in their simplicity and the fluid coordination they promote, which is essential for maintaining balance and stability as you age.

Tai Chi walking

Moving on to Tai Chi walking, which is a bit more dynamic, it's a wonderful way to enhance stability and mindfulness.

- Imagine you're walking on a line, heel to toe. Start with one foot forward, heel down first, and then roll through to the toe.

- As you step forward with the other foot, your heel touches down directly in front of the toe of your back foot, all while maintaining a smooth, continuous motion.

- Do this exercise for 30 seconds to one minute.

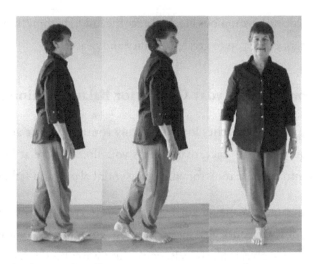

This methodical way of walking increases your control over your movements, which is crucial for preventing falls. It also forces you to concentrate on each step, which enhances mindfulness—a state where you're fully present in the moment, aware of your body and how it moves through space.

Another integral aspect of Tai Chi is the synchronisation of your breath with your movements. This practice is about more than just filling your lungs; it's about energising your entire body. For instance, when performing an arm raise, you would inhale slowly as your hands lift and exhale as they lower.

This not only helps to control the pace of your movements but also deepens your relaxation, making each session akin to a moving meditation. The deep breathing involved in Tai Chi increases lung capacity and circulation, and the focus on breath helps to centre your mind, reducing anxiety and promoting a state of calm.

Tai Chi is a gentle yet powerful way to enhance your physical balance through mindful movements and controlled breathing. It's particularly beneficial for seniors as it gently strengthens the muscles, reduces stress and improves mental focus and stability.

The slow, deliberate movements allow you to build strength and flexibility gradually, without straining your body. So, as you glide through each pose, remember that every gentle twist, every deliberate step, and every deep breath is a step toward a more balanced and harmonious life. Embrace the fluid, rhythmic motions of Tai Chi and let them guide you to greater stability and peace.

3.4 Incorporating Everyday Objects for Balance Training

Incorporating balance exercises into your daily routine doesn't always require specialised equipment. In fact, many items you already have at home can be transformed into effective tools for enhancing your balance and stability.

This approach not only makes your training more accessible but also adds a fun twist to your workouts, making them more enjoyable and engaging. Let's explore how simple objects like towels, books, and water bottles can become key components of your balance training regimen.

Using a Towel for Foot Grips

A common yet often overlooked aspect of maintaining balance is the strength of your foot muscles. Strong feet are the foundation upon which good balance is built, as they help you adjust and stabilise your body on various surfaces.

A simple towel can be a fantastic tool to help strengthen these muscles.

- Start by sitting comfortably in a chair with a flat towel placed on the floor in front of your feet. With your heels on the ground, use your toes to scrunch the towel towards you.

This motion engages the muscles in your feet and lower legs, which are crucial for maintaining balance. You can also perform this exercise while standing by placing one foot on the towel and trying to grip or lift the towel using only your toes, then alternating feet.

This not only strengthens the muscles but also enhances your foot's dexterity and control, which are essential for navigating uneven surfaces or quickly adjusting your stance to prevent a fall.

Balancing a Book on the Head

This next exercise might bring back memories of old charm school lessons, but balancing a book on your head is a fantastic way to improve your posture and stability.

Good posture is essential for good balance, as it aligns your body properly, allowing you to move more efficiently and with greater control.

- To start, choose a relatively hardcover book and place it on top of your head.

- Stand with your feet hip-width apart and your hands by your sides. Slowly start walking in a straight line, focusing on keeping the book balanced. Do this exercise for 30 seconds to a minute and gradually increase it as you get better.

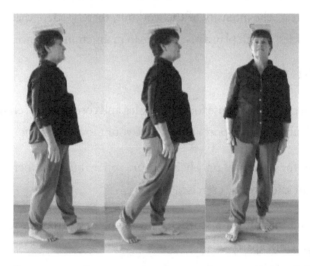

This exercise forces you to keep your head up and your spine straight, strengthening the postural muscles in your back and neck.

As you get more comfortable, you can try more challenging variations like turning your head from side to side or walking in a zigzag pattern. Not only does this exercise help improve your balance, but it also encourages you to be more aware of your body's positioning, which is crucial for maintaining stability.

Using Water Bottles as Weights

Water bottles can easily be used as makeshift weights for a range of exercises that build strength and enhance balance.

- Start with two water bottles of the same size and fill them with water to the desired weight.

- Holding a bottle in each hand, you can perform a variety of exercises like arm raises, side lifts, or even simple curls.

These movements help build upper body strength, which is important not only for balance but also for everyday activities such as carrying groceries or pushing open a heavy door.

Additionally, you can incorporate these improvised weights into your leg exercises. For instance, hold a water bottle in each hand while performing squats or lunges to increase the intensity of the workout, thereby strengthening your legs and core muscles, which play a pivotal role in maintaining balance.

Chair Assists for Squats

Squats are an excellent exercise for building leg and core strength, enhancing your lower body's ability to support and stabilise your movements.

Using a chair for squats not only helps ensure you maintain proper form but also adds a layer of safety to the exercise.

- Stand in front of a sturdy chair, facing away from it, with your feet hip-width apart.

- Extend your arms in front of you for balance. Slowly bend your knees and lower your hips as if you are about to sit down, then stop just before you reach the chair, hold for three to five seconds, then return to standing.

- The chair serves as a cue for how low you should go, preventing you from squatting too deeply, which can strain your knees.

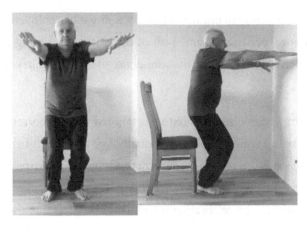

As you become more confident, you can reduce the reliance on the chair, using it only for occasional support or removing it altogether for a full squat. This exercise is particularly beneficial as it mimics the action of sitting down and standing up, which is a fundamental movement in daily life, ensuring you can perform such tasks with ease and stability.

Incorporating these everyday items into your balance training not only makes the exercises more accessible but also adds a playful element to your routine, making it more enjoyable.

Each of these tools—the towel, the book, the water bottles, and the chair—not only serve their primary functions but also become key players in your journey toward better balance and stability. By creatively using household items, you maintain your motivation to train regularly, which is essential for seeing continuous improvement in your balance and overall mobility.

So next time you pick up a towel, a book, or a water bottle, remember that they are not just simple objects but potential tools for enhancing your physical strength and stability, paving the way for a more active and independent life.

3.5 Building Confidence: Progress Tracking and Setting Goals

Navigating the pathway to improved balance is much like cultivating a garden; it requires patience, persistence, and a bit of daily nurture. Setting small, realistic goals is a cornerstone in building the confidence that will sustain you throughout this process.

These goals are your personal milestones, tailored to your current abilities and designed to expand your capabilities gradually. For instance, if balancing on one foot for five seconds is challenging, start there. Once you've mastered that, extend the time, or try the same exercise without any support. This approach not only keeps you motivated by celebrating incremental progress but also ensures that you are constantly challenging your abilities safely and sustainably.

Keeping a balance diary can be a transformative tool in your journey. It's your personal log where you jot down what exercises you did, how you felt about them, and any improvements or difficulties you encountered. Over time, this diary becomes a valuable record of your progress.

You might note that holding a balance pose feels easier than when you started, or that you can now do an exercise without holding onto a chair. These notes provide tangible proof of your progress and can be incredibly motivating. They also serve as a useful reference for adjusting your exercise routine. If a particular exercise consistently causes discomfort, it might be time to modify it or focus on others that bring better results.

Celebrating small successes is crucial in maintaining high spirits and motivation. Every achievement, no matter how minor it seems, is a step forward in your balance and overall health.

Did you manage an extra ten seconds in your balance pose today? That's fantastic! Celebrate these moments. Share them with friends or family, or reward yourself with a little treat. These celebrations reinforce positive feelings about your exercise routine, making it something you look forward to rather than a chore.

Lastly, the ability to adjust your goals as needed is an essential skill. Life is unpredictable, and new health considerations might arise, or you might find yourself progressing faster than expected. Both scenarios require adjustments to your goals. Regular check-ins with yourself, perhaps every month or at the end of a set program like this 21-day plan, can help determine if your current goals are still appropriate. If you've had a health setback, it might be necessary to scale back your exercises temporarily. Conversely, if you're finding the exercises too easy, it's time to increase their difficulty to continue challenging your balance. These adjustments keep your training effective and ensure that you're working at the optimal level for your health and abilities.

As you continue to track your progress, set and achieve new goals, and celebrate your successes, you'll find that your confidence in your balance and in yourself grows stronger. This chapter not only sets the foundation for such growth but also encourages a proactive and responsive approach to balance training, ensuring that it remains a rewarding and effective part of your life.

As we wrap up this chapter on building confidence through goal-setting and progress tracking, remember that each small step you take is a building block towards greater stability and independence. You're not just improving your balance; you're enhancing your overall quality of life, ensuring that each day can be met with vigour and confidence.

Let's carry this forward spirit into the next chapter, where we will explore intermediate balance challenges that await you. Here, you'll learn to refine the skills you've developed and push your boundaries safely and effectively.

CHAPTER 4

INTERMEDIATE BALANCE CHALLENGES

A H, YOU'VE MADE IT! It's wonderful to see you progressing and ready to step up your game with some intermediate challenges that will spice up your balance routine.

This chapter is designed to stretch your capabilities a bit further, pushing the boundaries of what you've already mastered and introducing you to exercises that mirror the dynamic and sometimes unpredictable scenarios of everyday life.

So, let's lace up those trainers, grab a sip of water, and dive right into the world of dynamic walking exercises. These aren't just about putting one foot in front of the other; they're about refining your reactions and boosting your confidence, no matter what the path ahead throws your way!

4.1 Dynamic Walking Exercises to Increase Stability

Heel-to-Toe Speed Variations

One of the foundational exercises for improving balance is the heel-to-toe walk. It's simple, effective, and wonderfully mimics the natural walking pattern. However, now that you're ready to challenge yourself further, let's add a twist—speed variations.

- Start at a slow pace, concentrating on placing your heel right in front of the toe of your opposite foot. Once you've got the hang of it, gradually increase your speed until you're walking as fast as you can while maintaining the heel-to-toe pattern.

- Do this exercise for one to two minutes and gradually build up overtime.

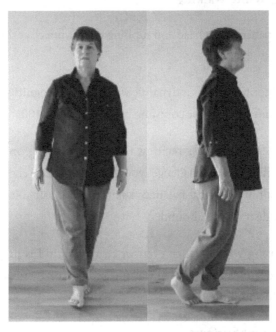

This acceleration forces your body to adjust quickly, enhancing your proprioceptive abilities—the fancy term for your body's ability to sense movement within the joints, muscles, and ligaments. It's a fantastic way to train your body to adapt to changes in pace, which you encounter while crossing streets or hurrying to answer the phone.

Direction Changes

Real life doesn't always allow us to move in a straight line; sometimes, it requires sudden twists and turns. Let's simulate that!

- While continuing your heel-to-toe walking, incorporate sudden yet controlled direction changes.

- Turn to your right, then back to your left, at random intervals. This exercise is not just about balance; it's about how quickly you can adapt to these changes without losing your footing. It sharpens your reaction time and prepares you for those unexpected moments, like dodging a wayward skateboard or navigating a crowded grocery store.

Multi-tasking While Walking

If you thought patting your head and rubbing your stomach at the same time was tough, try this!

- While continuing your dynamic walking, add a cognitive task. Start with something simple like counting backwards from 100.

- Ready for more? Try reciting a poem or carrying on a conversation. This multi-tasking challenges your brain to manage cognitive load while maintaining physical balance, a skill that's invaluable in everyday life where distractions abound.

It's about keeping your balance even when your mind is juggling multiple tasks—useful for times when you're walking and chatting with a friend or planning your day in your head.

Utilising Different Surfaces

To really test your balance skills, practice walking on different surfaces. Start with indoor surfaces like carpet or hardwood. Then, if you can, take it outside. Walk on grass, sand, or gravel. Each surface offers a new challenge, changing how your feet interact with the ground and requiring different levels of adjustment from your body.

This variety not only keeps the exercise interesting but also trains you to handle the diverse terrains you might encounter in your daily life, from the uneven pavement at the park to the soft, shifting sands of a beach.

These dynamic exercises are designed to reflect the real-world challenges you face every day. They keep your routine exciting and ensure that your balance training is comprehensive, covering not just static techniques but also those that require quick, responsive movements.

As you get better at these, you'll find yourself moving through life with greater ease and confidence, ready to take on whatever comes your way with a steady stride and a sure footing. So, enjoy the process, push your limits safely, and remember, that every step you take is a step toward a more balanced life.

Now, continue practising these dynamic walking exercises regularly. They are crucial for advancing your skills and ensuring that your balance is as dynamic and adaptable as the life you lead. Keep moving, keep adapting, and keep balancing!

4.2 Balance Walks with Obstacle Navigation

Imagine turning a little bit of your living space into a fun, challenging course that not only sharpens your balance but also spices up your daily exercise routine.

Setting up a safe, homemade obstacle course is like creating a mini-adventure park where you can refine your balance skills in a fun and controlled environment.

Start with simple items like cones, ropes, or even cushions to serve as obstacles. Arrange these items in a pathway that you can navigate through.

The key here is to ensure everything is securely placed to prevent any shifts that could lead to slips or trips. For instance, if using ropes, tape them down to the floor to keep them from moving underfoot. Cones are great because they're visible and stable, but make sure they're spaced in a way that challenges you without posing a risk.

Navigating your obstacle course safely requires a bit of technique, especially when you're stepping over or around obstacles. When approaching an obstacle, focus on maintaining a stable centre of gravity. This means keeping your body upright and using your arms for balance. When stepping over something, lift your foot higher than you feel is necessary. It might feel a bit exaggerated, but it ensures you clear the obstacle without catching your foot.

For stepping around objects, take slow, deliberate steps, making sure to plant your whole foot on the ground with each step, avoiding any half-steps or tiptoes, which can throw off your balance.

As your confidence grows, it's time to slowly increase the complexity of your course. Maybe add a few more cones, or arrange them in slightly more challenging patterns. Incorporate different heights or types of obstacles, like a small stool to step over or a soft pillow that tests your balance as you step on and off. Each new element should push you a bit further, helping build not just your physical balance but also your confidence in navigating through tricky paths. Remember, the goal is gradual improvement, so always update your course in small increments to ensure you continue to challenge yourself without becoming overwhelmed.

Recovery strategies are crucial, especially if you find yourself losing balance. One effective method is the controlled stop, where you feel yourself losing stability, stop moving immediately, and plant your feet firmly until you regain your balance.

Another handy technique is the catch step, where you use a quick, small step in the direction you're tipping to catch yourself. Both strategies can be practised during your obstacle course runs, providing not just a physical workout but also training your reflexes to react quickly and effectively in case of real-world stumbles.

Navigating through your custom obstacle course regularly not only keeps your routine engaging but also fine-tunes your abilities to handle real-life situations where good balance is crucial. Whether it's stepping over a puddle or manoeuvring around holiday decorations at home, the skills you develop here will make you adept at thinking on your feet—quite literally.

So, take this challenge in stride, enjoy the process, and watch as every step over a cone or rope translates into greater confidence and stability in your everyday life.

4.3 Moderate Tai Chi for Coordination and Control

As you continue to refine your balance and embrace new challenges, Tai Chi remains an invaluable ally. This ancient practice, rooted in martial arts, offers a unique blend of physical discipline and meditative calm, making it ideal for enhancing coordination and control.

At this stage, you might be familiar with basic Tai Chi forms, but let's take it a step further. Expanding on these, we'll explore more complex hand and arm movements that require a thoughtful, precise coordination. Imagine the grace of a conductor leading an orchestra; every movement is deliberate and flows into the next, creating a harmonious sequence. This is the essence of advanced Tai Chi forms.

Golden Rooster Stands on One Leg

Incorporating these advanced hand and arm movements, start with something like the "Golden Rooster Stands on One Leg." This pose not only challenges your balance but also demands great control over your limbs.

- As you stand on one leg, slowly raise the opposite knee while simultaneously lifting your arms to shoulder height, palms facing downward.

- The movement is slow, controlled, and deliberate, mirroring the precision needed to balance on one leg.

- As you hold this pose, focus on the stillness in movement, feeling how each muscle plays its role in maintaining your stability. Hold this pose for as long as possible and gradually hold it for longer as your balance improves.

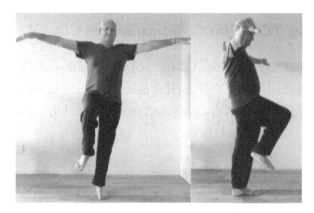

This exercise enhances your upper body coordination, crucial for tasks that require dexterity and precision, such as opening jars or rearranging items on a high shelf.

Bow Stance

Now, let's engage the lower body more intensely, which is pivotal for solidifying the foundation of your balance. Tai Chi offers various stances that involve deeper leg positions, such as the "Bow Stance," which strengthens your legs and improves your stability.

- To perform this, step forward with one foot and bend your knee, keeping your back leg straight, mimicking the stance of an archer.

- The depth of the stance can be adjusted according to your comfort and capability, but the goal is to challenge your leg muscles just enough to build strength without straining.

- Pair this stance with a slow, controlled arm movement, like pushing the palms forward as if gently pushing against resistance, to integrate the upper and lower body in one fluid motion.

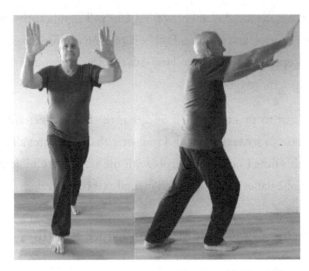

The flow between movements in Tai Chi is where the magic really happens. This continuous, fluid motion is not just about aesthetics; it plays a crucial role in improving your dynamic balance and agility. Think of it as a dance, where each step and turn flows seamlessly into the next.

Practising this flow helps your body learn to adjust smoothly to changing positions, which is especially useful in preventing falls. If you stumble or trip, your body is better equipped to flow into a recovery position naturally, reducing the risk of injury.

Lastly, the synchronisation of breath with movement in Tai Chi transforms the practice from mere physical exercise to a meditative experience. This deep awareness of breath helps to centre your mind, enhancing focus and reducing stress.

As you move through each form, coordinate your inhalations and exhalations with your movements. For instance, as you expand your arms outward in a gesture of opening, inhale deeply, filling your lungs and expanding your chest; as you withdraw your arms, exhale slowly, letting the air carry away tension and fatigue.

This practice of breath synchronisation not only improves respiratory efficiency but also deepens the meditative aspect of Tai Chi, making each session a holistic experience of physical exercise and mental relaxation.

Embracing these advanced elements of Tai Chi will significantly enhance your coordination, control, and balance. Each session is an opportunity to refine your techniques, deepen your breath, and smooth the flow of movements, contributing to a stronger, more agile you.

As you continue to practice, you'll find that the benefits extend beyond the physical, fostering a sense of calm and resilience that permeates all areas of your life. So, take this time to connect deeply with the art of Tai Chi, letting it guide you to a state of balance that is as much mental as it is physical.

4.4 Integrating Light Weights into Balance Routines

Incorporating light weights into your balance routine is like adding a pinch of spice to a favourite dish—it enhances the flavour, bringing out the best in all the ingredients.

Similarly, adding weights to your exercises can significantly amplify their benefits, helping to strengthen the muscles that keep you stable and upright. However, like any good recipe, success lies in using the right amount and handling it properly to avoid any mishaps.

Let's start by talking about how to select the appropriate weight sizes for your exercises. It's crucial to choose weights that challenge you without causing strain or risking injury. A good rule of thumb is to start light, especially if you're new to using weights. For most, this might mean beginning with one or two-pound hand weights. As you grow more comfortable and your strength improves, you can gradually increase your weight.

Always listen to your body—if an exercise feels too easy, it might be time to go a bit heavier, but if you start to compromise your form to lift the weight, it's too heavy.

Safe handling and positioning of weights are paramount. When lifting weights, ensure you do so with controlled movements to avoid jerking, which can lead to injuries. For example, when doing arm exercises, keep your wrists straight and your elbows slightly bent to prevent strain. Always lift using your arms and shoulders, not your back.

It's also wise to perform these exercises standing on a non-slip surface to ensure stability, especially when you're adding the challenge of weights to your balance exercises. Proper posture is your best friend here; keep your spine neutral, your chest open, and your gaze forward to maintain balance and ensure effective form throughout each exercise.

Leg curls

Let's delve into some specific exercises that incorporate light weights, beginning with the legs. Leg curls or lifts, for instance, are excellent for strengthening the muscles at the back of your thighs, which are crucial for maintaining balance.

- Try this: stand behind your chair, using it for support, if needed.

- Hold a weight in each hand, letting them hang naturally at your sides.

- Slowly bend one knee, lifting your heel towards your buttock as comfortably as possible, then lower it back down. Repeat this movement five times before switching legs.

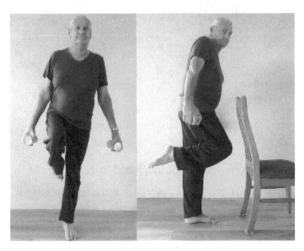

This exercise not only strengthens your hamstrings but also engages your core and improves your balance as you lift and lower your leg.

Overhead press

Now, for your upper body, combining strength exercises like overhead presses or lateral raises with balance challenges can be particularly effective.

- Here's an idea: stand on one foot – use your chair for support if needed – while performing an overhead press.

- Hold a light weight in each hand, start with your arms bent, weights at shoulder height, and press them upwards until your arms are straight but not locked, hold for five seconds. Bring them back down slowly. Repeat five to ten times.

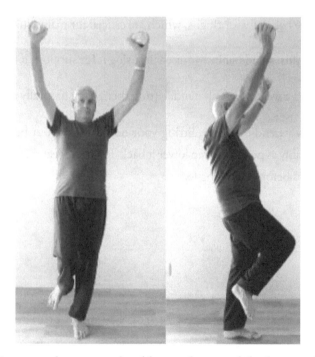

This exercise strengthens your shoulders and arms while the act of balancing on one foot works your core and stabiliser muscles, making it a dual-benefit movement.

Weighted Twist

Finally, let's focus on using weights to enhance core stability, which is essential for overall balance.

A great exercise here is the weighted twist.

- Hold a single lightweight with both hands in front of you, elbows bent.

- Stand with your feet hip-width apart. Slowly rotate your torso to the right, keeping your hips facing forward, then rotate to the left, holding each side for five to ten seconds.

- Repeat five to ten times.

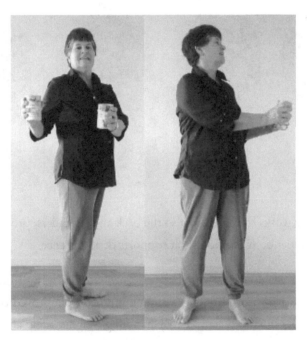

This movement engages the core muscles deeply, enhancing their strength and endurance, which are vital for maintaining balance.

Standing Paddle Row

Alternatively, try the standing paddle row, which mimics the motion of rowing a boat.

- Stand with feet hip-width apart, a weight in each hand.

- Bend your knees slightly, hinge forward at your hips, and pull the weights back towards your hips, elbows going behind you, then extend your arms back out. Hold for as long as possible.

- Repeat five to ten times.

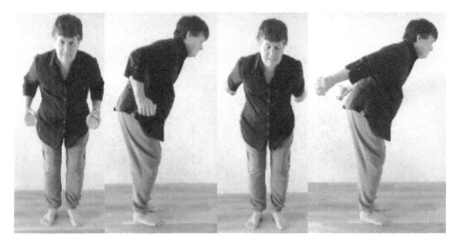

This not only works the core but also the back and shoulders, providing a comprehensive upper body workout that supports better balance.

Incorporating weights into your balance routine offers a multitude of benefits, from increased muscle strength and endurance to improved coordination and, ultimately, enhanced stability. By handling weights safely and integrating them into various exercises, you create a more robust and effective workout that supports your everyday activities. Whether you're carrying groceries, lifting a grandchild, or simply navigating busy streets, the strength and stability gained from these exercises help ensure that you can do so with confidence and ease.

4.5 Partner Exercises for Fun and Functionality

Imagine turning your balance practice into a shared activity that not only enhances your physical health but also strengthens your social connections.

Working out with a partner adds a layer of fun and functionality to your routine, making the exercises not just more enjoyable but also more effective. You can encourage each other, share laughs, and celebrate progress together, all while improving your balance and coordination.

Let's explore some partner exercises that are perfect for doubling the fun and the benefits.

Mirroring Exercises

One of the most engaging partner exercises is mirroring, where one person leads by performing a movement, and the other follows, trying to mirror the movement as closely as possible.

This can include anything from simple arm raises to more complex sequences involving stepping or bending. The key here is the interaction and the challenge of copying movements accurately, which greatly enhances your coordination and the ability to maintain balance in response to visual cues.

As you and your partner switch roles between leader and follower, you not only work on your physical balance but also develop a deeper level of communication and connection, making the exercise both a physical and social activity. It's like a dance where each movement brings you closer, not just in steps but in sync.

Assisted Stretching

Stretching is vital for maintaining flexibility, which in turn supports your balance. When you engage in assisted stretching with a partner, you can achieve more than when stretching alone.

Your partner can help you maintain a pose longer or reach a bit further, pushing you gently to extend your range of motion safely.

For example, one effective stretch involves one person sitting with legs extended forward while the other gently presses on the soles to deepen the stretch. This mutual support not only helps improve your flexibility but also ensures you both practice safe stretching techniques, reducing the risk of overextending and injury.

Assisted stretching can be a deeply relaxing and trust-building activity, as you rely on each other to respect limits and provide just the right amount of pressure to aid in stretching.

Balance Support Drills

Using each other for support, you can engage in balance drills that might be too challenging to attempt alone. An enjoyable and effective exercise is the back-to-back stand.

Stand with your backs touching and slowly lean away from each other, using each other's weight as a counterbalance. Try to find the point where you are both leaning but still stable, holding the position as long as you can.

This exercise not only helps strengthen your core muscles, which are essential for good balance but also requires a high degree of coordination and trust between partners, enhancing your ability to work together and support each other.

Fun Competitive Challenges

To add an element of light-hearted competition, try setting up challenges like balance beam walking contests or tandem walking drills where you both walk heel-to-toe while linked arm in arm.

These challenges can be a fun way to test your skills against each other, providing motivation to improve and a few laughs along the way. Competing in a friendly manner keeps the mood upbeat and makes the time spent exercising fly by.

It's not just about who can balance the longest, but about sharing moments of joy and encouragement, celebrating each other's successes, and sometimes, amusing missteps.

Engaging in these partner exercises transforms your balance practice from a solitary activity into a shared endeavour that brings a multitude of benefits. It enhances your physical coordination, builds social bonds, and injects a sense of joy and playfulness into your workouts. By incorporating these exercises into your routine, you not only improve your own balance but also contribute to a healthier, happier partnership, whether with a spouse, a friend, or a family member.

So, grab a partner and make your next workout a joint adventure that's twice as effective and twice as enjoyable.

As we wrap up this chapter on intermediate balance challenges, remember that the journey to better balance is one best shared. The exercises and techniques explored here are designed to push your limits, enhance your coordination, and bring a bit of fun into your routine.

Looking ahead, the next chapter will introduce advanced balance techniques that will further refine your skills and provide you with the tools to tackle even more complex balance tasks. Keep moving forward, keep challenging yourself, and most importantly, keep enjoying every step of the process.

CHAPTER 5

ADVANCED BALANCE TECHNIQUES

W HEN YOU FIRST BEGAN this balance-enhancing adventure, it might have felt like tiptoeing across a narrow beam high above the ground—exciting, yes, but a tad intimidating! Now, here you are, ready to level up and tackle some advanced techniques. It's like you've been handed the keys to a more expansive playground, where each new challenge is a doorway to better stability, strength, and agility.

So, let's roll up our sleeves and dive into some sophisticated balance exercises that will not only challenge you but also bring a whole new level of fun and functionality to your daily routines.

5.1 Advanced Strength and Balance Combinations

Integration of Multi-Directional Movements

One of the most exhilarating ways to enhance your balance and overall mobility is to incorporate multi-directional movements into your exercises. Imagine the freedom and ease you'll feel as your body learns to swiftly and smoothly navigate in any direction, just like a skilled dancer or martial artist.

Lunges combined with reaches or twists

Let's start with a dynamic exercise: lunges combined with reaches or twists.

- Here's how to do it: step forward into a lunge, making sure your front knee is aligned with your ankle and your back knee is slightly bent towards the floor.

- As you settle into the lunge, extend your arms and twist your torso towards the leg that is forward. Hold for as long as possible.

- Repeat five to ten times.

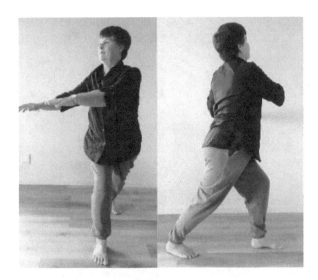

This not only challenges your balance but also strengthens your legs, core, and the flexibility of your spine. The beauty of this exercise lies in its mimicry of real-life movements—like reaching for a high shelf while stepping around an obstacle. It's functional fitness that prepares you for the unpredictability of everyday life.

Dynamic Balance on Unstable Surfaces

Now, let's take your balance training to an exciting new level by introducing unstable surfaces. Using tools like balance cushions or BOSU balls, you can significantly enhance your body's stability and core control.

- Here's an exercise to try: stand on a BOSU ball, if you don't have one use a couch cushion with your feet hip-width apart. The soft, unstable surface will immediately engage your core and leg muscles, which kick into gear trying to stabilise your body.

- From this position, perform arm raises or side bends, and hold each position for five to ten seconds. Each movement requires your muscles to adapt quickly to maintain balance, intensifying the workout and dramatically improving your core strength and stability.

- Repeat three to five times.

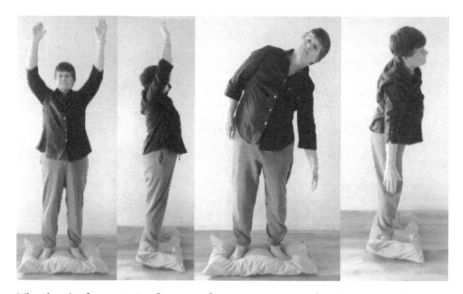

This kind of training is fantastic for preparing you for situations where the ground isn't quite as steady—think of walking on a sandy beach or a snowy path.

Strength-Building with Functional Movements

Squat-to-stand exercise

Incorporating functional movements into your balance training enhances both strength and practical daily skills. A great example is the squat-to-stand exercise using a chair.

- Start by sitting in a chair with your feet flat on the floor. Lean forward slightly and stand up without using your hands.

- To add to the challenge, hold a lightweight in each hand as you stand.

- Once you're up, slowly sit back down. Repeat this movement five to ten times.

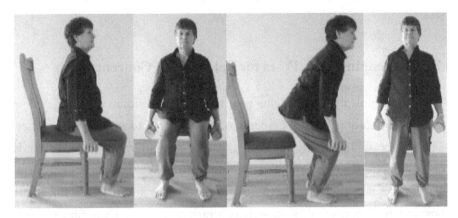

This exercise strengthens your thighs, hips, and buttocks while also improving your ability to perform one of the most common daily movements—rising from and sitting in a chair. It's about building strength through movements that are part of your everyday life, making them easier and safer.

Circuit Training for Balance and Strength

Circuit training is a fantastic way to keep your workout exciting and challenging. It involves moving quickly from one exercise to another, which keeps your heart rate up and challenges your muscles in various ways.

Set up a circuit that includes a variety of balance and strength exercises, like the ones mentioned above, along with others you've learned along the way. For instance, you might start with lunges and twists, move to the BOSU ball for some dynamic balance work, then do a series of functional squats, and finish with a light jog or walk-in place. The quick pace and variety not only makes the time fly by but also significantly boost your endurance and agility, making you stronger and more balanced in every sense.

Engaging in these advanced balance techniques is about pushing the boundaries of what you can achieve, exploring how far you can stretch your abilities, and revelling in the newfound strength and stability that come from your efforts. Each session is an opportunity to explore, play, and refine your skills, ensuring that as you move through your day-to-day life, each step is taken with confidence and grace. So, embrace these challenges, enjoy the process, and continue to build that strong, balanced body that carries you through every adventure life throws your way.

5.2 Challenging Yoga Poses for Balance and Concentration

When you think about enhancing your balance and concentration, yoga offers some incredible opportunities, especially as you progress to more advanced poses. The beauty of challenging yoga poses, particularly inversions like headstands or handstands, lies in their ability to transform your physical and mental state. These poses take your practice to new heights—quite literally! Let's talk about how to safely approach these inversions, which are not just about flipping your perspective but also about strengthening your upper body, engaging your core, and, importantly, building an incredible amount of balance.

Inversions like the headstand or handstand bring a playful yet profound dimension to your yoga practice. Before attempting these, it's crucial to build a strong foundation. Start with less intense inversions such as the Dolphin pose or a supported headstand using a wall. These preparatory poses help you build the necessary upper body strength and confidence. When you're ready to try a full inversion, ensure you do so in a safe environment—free from clutter and with plenty of space. Using a wall for support can be immensely helpful. Remember, the key is to move into these poses slowly and with control, using your hands and arms to stabilise your balance as you lift your legs up. Engaging your core is crucial here; it helps you maintain stability and protects your lower back.

Transitioning smoothly in your yoga practice enhances not only the flow of your session but also your balance and concentration. Flow sequences, particularly those that move from one challenging pose to another like from Warrior III to Half Moon pose, require a deep focus and a strong connection with your body.

Warrior III

- Warrior III: While seated on a chair hinge at the hips with one leg extended fully behind you and arms outstretched in front, forming a 'T' with your body. Hold for five to ten seconds and repeat five times.

- This pose tests your balance and strengthens your legs and core.

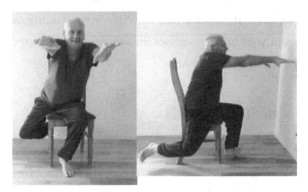

Advanced yoga poses often require the aid of props, and knowing how to use them effectively can significantly enhance your practice. Props like yoga blocks or straps are not just aids but tools to deepen your practice and perform poses correctly. For instance, in poses where balance and flexibility are challenged, such as in the Revolved Triangle pose, a block can be used to support your hand if it doesn't comfortably reach the floor. This allows you to open your chest fully and twist deeper without compromising your balance or alignment. Similarly, straps can be used in balancing poses where your hands may not reach your feet, maintaining alignment and helping you gradually deepen into the pose without strain.

Focusing on your breath is essential in any yoga practice, but it becomes even more critical when performing advanced poses. Controlled, mindful breathing helps to steady your balance, calm your mind, and maintain focus. Each inhalation and exhalation should be deep and even, especially when holding a challenging pose. This not only keeps you steady but also infuses a meditative quality into your practice, turning each session into a serene flow of movements and breath. The continuous focus on breath keeps you anchored in the present moment, fully engaged with each movement and adjustment, enhancing both your physical balance and mental clarity.

Exploring these advanced yoga techniques brings a new layer of depth to your balance training. It's about pushing the boundaries of what you can achieve and discovering a profound sense of strength and stability. As you integrate these challenging poses and techniques into your practice, you'll notice not just improvements in your physical balance, but also a greater calmness and focus in your daily life. So, embrace these advanced exercises with enthusiasm and patience, and watch as your yoga practice evolves into an even more rewarding journey of balance, strength, and tranquillity.

5.3 Pilates with Stability Balls

Incorporating stability balls into your Pilates routine opens up a new dimension of core strengthening and balance enhancement that you might find both challenging and exhilarating. Let's explore some advanced core exercises that utilise the stability ball, starting with the roll-outs and pikes. These movements require a good deal of core strength and stability, which are essential for maintaining balance and overall functional fitness.

Roll-out pose

- Kneel on a mat with the stability/swiss ball in front of you (if you don't have a ball, roll up a towel and use that).

- Place your forearms on the ball/towel, hands clasped together. Slowly roll the ball away from you, extending your body as you go, keeping your back straight and your core tight.

- Then, using your core muscles, pull the ball back towards you, returning to your starting position. This exercise engages your entire core, improving your control and stability.

- Repeat five to ten times.

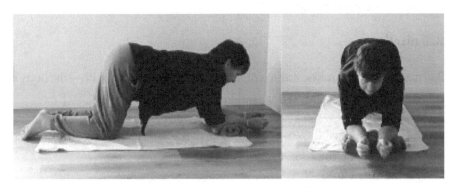

Pikes

Moving on to pikes, this exercise begins in a similar position to the roll-out but adds an element of hip elevation.

- Start in a push-up position with your feet on the stability/swiss ball (or a rolled-up towel if you don't have a ball).

- Keeping your legs straight and your core engaged, use your abdominal muscles to lift your hips towards the ceiling, pulling the ball towards your arms, then lowering back into a plank position.

- Hold this position for as long as possible and gradually increase as you get stronger.

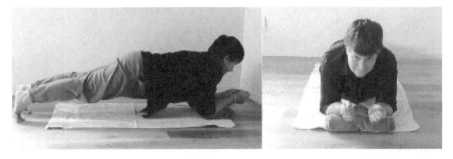

This movement not only challenges your core but also your shoulder stability and balance. As you perform these exercises, focus on maintaining control and balance, which are key to executing them correctly and safely.

Now let's turn our attention to exercises that challenge your balance while seated or lying on the stability ball.

Ball marches

Ball marches are a fantastic way to enhance your proprioceptive skills—the body's ability to sense movement, action, and location.

- Sit on the stability/swiss ball (or a chair if you don't have a ball) with your feet flat on the floor.

- Slowly lift one foot off the ground, hold for five to ten seconds, then switch to the other foot.

- Repeat five to ten times.

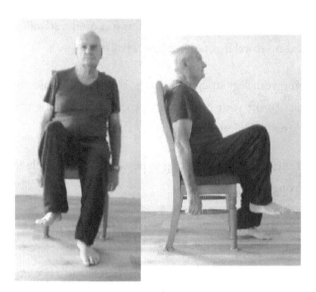

As you get more comfortable, you can increase the challenge by extending your leg straight out or adding arm movements.

Hip lift

Another great exercise is the hip lift.

- Lie down on the floor with your knees bent and feet flat on the floor.

- Push through your feet to lift your hips towards the ceiling, forming a straight line from your shoulders to your knees, then slowly lower back down.

- Hold for 10 to 30 seconds. Repeat five times.

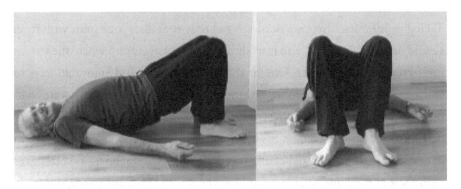

These exercises not only improve your core strength but also challenge your balance in a dynamic way, making everyday activities easier and safer.

Integrating resistance bands with stability balls can provide a comprehensive workout that targets multiple muscle groups simultaneously. For example, try wrapping a resistance band around the bottom of your feet while sitting on the stability ball with the ends of the band in each hand. Perform exercises like chest presses or rows by pulling against the resistance band while maintaining your balance on the ball. This combination not only strengthens your arms and chest but also engages your core and improves your balance as you stabilise yourself on the moving ball. It's a full-body workout that enhances your strength, stability, and coordination.

Safety is paramount when performing exercises on a stability ball, especially when incorporating resistance bands or additional weights. Always ensure you choose the right size ball for your height and check it for any signs of wear or damage before use. When sitting or lying on the ball, make sure your weight is evenly distributed and the ball is stable. Use a mat to prevent the ball from slipping, and if you're new to these exercises, have a chair or a wall nearby for support. As with any exercise routine, listen to your body and modify the movements to suit your fitness level and balance capabilities. By following these safety guidelines, you can enjoy the benefits of stability ball exercises safely and effectively, pushing your balance and core strength to new heights without risking injury.

5.4 Outdoor Balance Activities for Varied Terrain

Taking your balance exercises outdoors not only revitalises your spirit with fresh air and natural beauty but also introduces you to a playground where the terrain itself becomes your trainer. One of the most enriching and enjoyable ways to enhance your balance outdoors is through trail walking that incorporates natural obstacles. Imagine stepping over a fallen log or maneuvering around rocky paths—each step you take on these uneven surfaces challenges your balance in dynamic ways that a flat, predictable gym floor simply cannot offer. As you engage with these natural obstacles, your ankles, knees, and hips learn to adapt quickly to unexpected changes in the environment, significantly improving your agility and reaction times. This type of walking not only boosts your physical balance but also sharpens your mental focus as you must constantly be aware of the next foot placement.

Navigating different types of ground surfaces is another thrilling challenge. Whether it's the give of a sandy beach, the irregularity of a gravel path, or the soft cushioning of a grassy field, each surface brings its own set of challenges and benefits. For instance, sand is excellent for building the small stabiliser muscles in your feet and ankles, which are crucial for balance. Walking on grass, meanwhile, can be surprisingly tiring for the muscles, providing a good workout because the soft surface absorbs more energy. Gravel paths train you to maintain stability even when the ground isn't solid, enhancing your confidence and skills in preventing slips and falls. Techniques for maintaining balance on these surfaces include maintaining a lower centre of gravity by bending your knees slightly and using your arms for additional balance, much like a tightrope walker uses their balancing pole.

Good navigational skills are essential when you're moving through varied outdoor environments. This involves not just knowing the route but also being able to read the terrain and adjust your movements accordingly. Visual scanning is a vital skill here; it involves constantly looking ahead and around, not just at your feet, to anticipate obstacles or changes in the terrain. This proactive scanning helps you plan your movements in advance, making adjustments in stride length or speed as needed, which is crucial for safe and efficient travel through natural landscapes. Such skills are immensely useful, not just on nature trails but also in urban settings where uneven pavement or unexpected obstacles can pose a risk.

Lastly, let's talk about using natural elements as part of your exercise routine. The outdoors is filled with opportunities to enhance your workout. For instance, a sturdy tree stump can be perfect for step-ups or balancing exercises. Benches are great for incline push-ups or tricep dips. Even a low branch can be used for modified pull-ups. Using these elements not only adds variety to your routine but also makes the workout more enjoyable. It's about being creative and viewing the natural landscape not just as a backdrop for your exercise routine but as an integral part of it. This approach not only enhances the physical challenge but also keeps the workouts engaging and fun, fostering a deeper connection with the environment and a greater appreciation for your body's capabilities within it.

Engaging in outdoor balance activities offers a refreshing twist to conventional balance training. It challenges you in new and unexpected ways, providing not only physical benefits but also mental and emotional rejuvenation. So next time you step outside, look at your surroundings with fresh eyes and see a world of opportunities to test and improve your balance and stability. Whether it's a quiet forest trail, a bustling city park, or even your backyard, each space has unique features that can help you push your balance abilities further, making every step a new discovery in your ongoing adventure of staying active and balanced.

5.5 Creating a Personalised Advanced Balance Routine

When it comes to enhancing your balance and overall stability, a one-size-fits-all approach just won't cut it. Each of us has unique needs, capabilities, and goals, making it essential to tailor your balance routine to fit your personal journey. Let's start by assessing where you stand—literally and figuratively. A thorough assessment can shed light on your strengths and pinpoint areas where you might need some extra attention. For instance, you might find that while your forward balance is quite strong, lateral movements might be a bit shaky. This insight directs the customisation of your routine, ensuring that it addresses your specific needs and helps you build a more rounded skill set.

Setting goals is not just about reaching a benchmark; it's about crafting milestones that keep you motivated and engaged. Whether it's perfecting a specific yoga pose that challenges your balance or completing an outdoor trail that includes navigating various terrains, these goals should stretch your abilities and inspire continuous improvement. Remember, these goals should be challenging yet achievable; they need to push you but also be realistic enough to keep frustration at bay. Achieving these goals brings a sense of accomplishment that fuels your motivation to set and reach even higher milestones.

Variety is the spice of life, and this holds especially true for your exercise routine. Incorporating a range of exercises prevents your workout from becoming monotonous and helps avoid hitting a plateau. It's crucial to periodically introduce new challenges that keep your body guessing and adapting. For instance, if you've been practising static balance exercises, why not shake things up by adding some dynamic movements that mimic everyday activities? Or, if you've been working indoors, take your routine outside to navigate different surfaces. These changes make your practice more comprehensive and engaging, ensuring that both your body and mind remain active and challenged.

Tracking your progress is key to understanding how well your routine is working for you. Keeping an exercise journal or using fitness apps can provide valuable feedback on your improvements and highlight areas that might need more attention. This ongoing record not only serves as a motivational tool—showing you just how far you've come—but also helps in fine-tuning your routine. Based on your progress, you might decide to intensify certain exercises or maybe scale back others. This kind of adjustment is crucial for maintaining a balance routine that continuously supports your growth and adaptation.

In summary, developing a personalised advanced balance routine is about under-standing and addressing your unique needs, setting compelling goals, embracing variety to stay engaged, and keeping track of your progress to fine-tune your approach. Each step you take should feel tailored just for you, ensuring that as you advance, your balance does too, supporting a richer, more active lifestyle.

As we wrap up this exploration of advanced balance techniques, remember that the journey to enhanced stability is ongoing. The skills you've developed here pave the way for not just better physical health but also a deeper understanding of your body's capabilities and needs. Continue to challenge yourself, stay curious, and embrace each new step with confidence. Up next, we'll explore how to maintain these skills over the long term, ensuring that your hard-earned balance is a lasting asset in your pursuit of an active, fulfilling life.

CHAPTER 6

DEVELOPING CORE STRENGTH AND FLEXIBILITY

I MAGINE YOUR BODY AS the foundation of a house. Just like a house needs a solid foundation to stay upright and withstand whatever comes its way, your body needs a strong core to maintain balance and move with ease. Whether you're picking up a grandchild, reaching for a top shelf, or simply walking to the mailbox, a strong and flexible core is your secret weapon to moving with confidence and avoiding injuries. In this chapter, we dive into exercises that fortify this central support system of your body, enhancing both your posture and your ability to stay balanced on your own two feet.

6.1 Core-Building Exercises for Better Posture and Balance

Plank Variations

Starting with planks might sound a bit daunting—after all, it's an exercise that even athletes treat with respect! But don't worry, you'll be beginning with modified versions that are much gentler on your body while still being wonderfully effective. Using a sturdy chair or even a wall, you can perform a standing plank that engages your core muscles without the strain of getting down on the floor.

- Stand facing the wall, about an arm's length away. Place your palms on the wall at shoulder height, then walk your feet back until your body forms a straight line from your head to your heels, just like a diagonal plank.

- Hold this position for as long as possible, pulling your naval towards your spine to deeply engage your core.

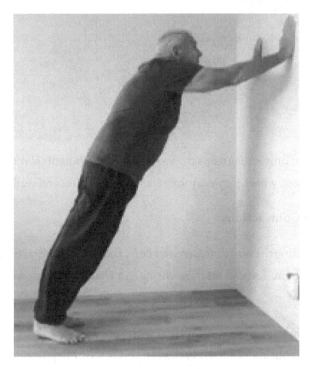

Over time, as your strength builds, you can gradually progress to more traditional planks on the ground, starting on your knees and eventually, perhaps, moving to your toes.

Bridges for Lower Back and Core

Now, let's get down to one of the best exercises for your lower back and core—the bridge.

- Lie on your back with your knees bent and feet flat on the floor, hip-width apart.

- Place your arms at your sides with palms down. Push through your heels to lift your hips off the floor, creating a straight line from your knees to your shoulders.

- Squeeze your buttocks and engage your core as you lift, holding the position for five to ten seconds before gently lowering back down. Repeat five to ten times.

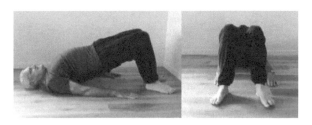

This move not only strengthens the lower back and abdominal muscles but also works the glutes, which play a critical role in your balance and walking abilities.

Abdominal Contractions

For strengthening the very centre of your core, abdominal contractions are simple yet super effective. You can do these sitting in a chair or lying down—whichever suits you best.

- If you're in a chair, sit upright with your feet flat on the ground. Contract your abdominal muscles as if you're trying to pull your belly button back towards the spine. Hold this squeeze for five to ten seconds, then release.

- Repeat five times, focusing on the tightening and relaxing, which strengthens your core muscles and enhances your posture.

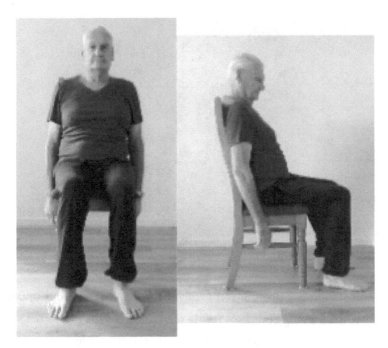

- If you're lying down, the process is the same, and you can place your hands under your lower back for additional support if needed.

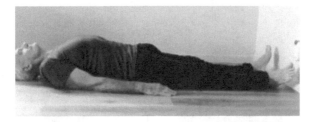

Rotation Movements

Lastly, let's add some rotation movements to improve the flexibility of your torso, which will help you in everyday activities, especially those involving turning or reaching across. Seated or standing, you can perform gentle torso rotations to build strength and increase flexibility.

- If seated, sit upright and slowly turn your upper body to the right, aiming to look over your shoulder, hold for five to ten seconds, then return to the centre and repeat on the left side. Repeat five to ten times.

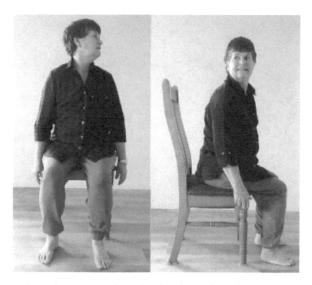

- If standing, keep your feet firmly planted and rotate your upper body while keeping your hips facing forward. hold for five to ten seconds, then return to the centre and repeat on the other side. Repeat five to ten times.

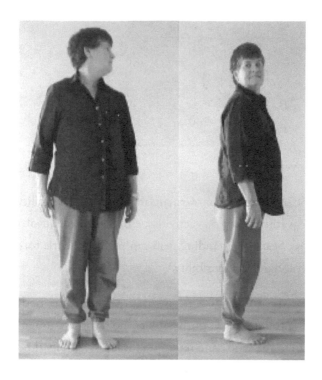

These rotations engage not just your core but also the muscles around your spine, enhancing your overall flexibility and balance.

By integrating these exercises into your daily routine, you're not just working towards a stronger core; you're setting the stage for better balance, smoother movements, and a healthier back. Each exercise has been chosen for its effectiveness and ease of adaptation, ensuring that you can progress at your own pace, safely and enjoyably. Remember, the core is at the centre of all you do—it supports every bend, every twist, and every step. Strengthening it is one of the best decisions you can make for your overall health and mobility. So take these exercises, tailor them to your needs, and start building a stronger foundation today.

6.2 Flexibility Routines to Aid in Movement and Stability

Imagine how a well-oiled hinge moves so smoothly, almost effortlessly—that's how your joints can feel when you integrate effective flexibility routines into your daily regimen. Starting with dynamic stretches, these are not your old-school hold-and-stretch routines. Instead, think of them as your body's way of easing into movement, warming up the muscles and joints in a way that prepares them for the activities ahead. Dynamic stretches are characterised by their active, controlled movements that improve blood flow and flexibility, which are essential for maintaining your mobility and stability.

Leg Swings and Arm Circles

One of the simplest yet most effective dynamic stretches involves leg swings.

- Hold onto the back of a sturdy chair or a countertop for balance and gently swing one leg forward and backward.

This movement stretches the hamstring and hip flexor muscles while also warming them up. Another great dynamic stretch is arm circles,

- Extend your arms straight out to the sides, at shoulder height and slowly rotate them in large circles.

This helps loosen up the shoulders and improves the range of motion, which is fantastic for any activities that involve lifting or reaching. Incorporating these types of stretches into your morning routine or before any exercise program not only preps your muscles and joints for movement but also decreases the risk of injuries, ensuring you can continue your activities with ease and comfort.

Now, transitioning from the warm-up phase of your routine, let's focus on static stretching, which is best performed at the end of your exercise session. Static stretches involve extending a muscle to its fullest and holding it in that position for a period, usually about 20-30 seconds. These stretches are crucial because they help maintain the flexibility gained during your workout and can significantly aid in your muscle recovery, reducing soreness. A focus on major muscle groups involved in balance—such as the hamstrings, quadriceps, and calves—is essential.

Hamstring Stretch

- For instance, a simple yet effective stretch for your hamstrings involves sitting on the floor with your legs extended straight, slowly bending forward at the waist, and reaching for your toes. Hold for as long as possible, repeat five times.

- If reaching your toes feels too challenging, no worries—just reach as far as you comfortably can. Over time, you'll notice your flexibility improving.

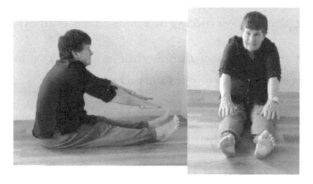

Incorporating flexibility exercises into your daily activities can also enhance your routine and ensure you stay limber throughout the day, not just during your workout times. For example, while watching TV, you can perform seated ankle rotations or neck stretches during commercials. These small movements keep your joints from getting stiff and improve blood circulation, which is especially important if you find yourself sitting for long periods. Another tip is to use moments like waiting for the kettle to boil or the microwave to beep as opportunities for quick stretches, like reaching up to stretch your sides or doing calf raises while holding onto the counter.

Partner Stretching Options

Involving a friend or family member in your stretching routine can not only make the experience more enjoyable but also more effective. Partner stretching allows for a deeper stretch as your partner can help support your body in a position that might be difficult to achieve alone.

For instance, a partner can assist in a quadricep stretch by holding your ankle while you focus on balancing with your other leg. This can help you achieve a deeper muscle stretch safely, enhancing your flexibility more effectively than when stretching alone. Always ensure that both you and your partner communicate openly during these exercises to avoid any discomfort or injury, and remember, the goal is gentle enhancement, not pushing each other into painful ranges of motion.

Through these flexibility routines, whether performed solo or with a partner, you're not just working towards greater flexibility but also ensuring that your body remains capable and ready for the many joys of movement. Each stretch, each bend, and each twist enhances your body's ability to move with grace and stability, keeping you active and agile as you navigate through your day with ease. Remember, flexibility is not just about touching your toes; it's about expanding your range of motion to embrace a fuller, more vibrant life.

6.3 Low-Impact Yoga Poses for Seniors

Yoga can be a wonderful addition to your life, especially as you age. It's not just about twisting into pretzel shapes; it's more about finding balance, stretching gently, and building strength in a way that's kind to your body. What's fantastic about yoga is its adaptability. Regardless of your fitness level or mobility, there are ways to modify yoga poses so everyone can benefit. Especially with the use of a chair, yoga becomes accessible to all. Chair yoga is a wonderful variant of traditional yoga as it allows you to perform various poses with the added support and stability of a chair. This can be particularly helpful if you're concerned about balance or if standing for extended periods is uncomfortable.

Seated Forward Bend

Let's explore some chair yoga poses that are excellent for seniors. A seated forward bend, for instance, is a great way to stretch your back and hamstrings gently.

- Sitting on a chair, keep your feet flat on the floor and slowly bend forward from your hips, extending your hands towards your feet. Hold for 20 – 30 seconds.

This movement helps lengthen the spine and relieve tension in the back, promoting flexibility and easing pain or discomfort.

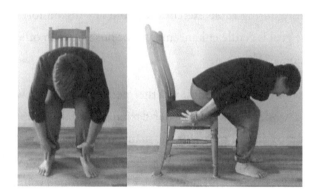

Chair Warrior

Another beneficial chair yoga pose is the chair warrior.

- While seated, simply extend one leg back, keeping the other bent in front of you, and raise your arms towards the ceiling. Hold for 20 – 30 seconds.

This pose strengthens your legs and improves your upper body flexibility, enhancing your overall posture and balance.

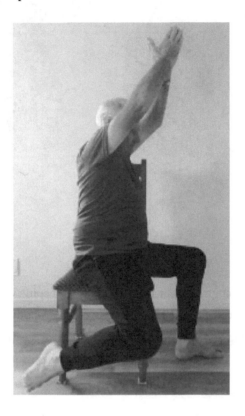

Tree Pose

Speaking of balance, yoga offers specific poses known for improving this vital skill. The tree pose, for example, is a popular balance-enhancing pose that can be modified for varying mobility levels.

- Using a chair for support (only if needed), stand and place the sole of one foot on the inside of the opposite thigh or calf (never on the knee), balancing on one leg. Hold for 20 – 30 seconds, then switch sides.

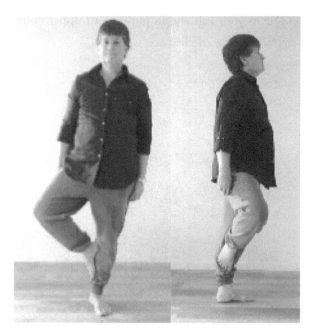

This pose helps strengthen your thighs, ankles, and spine while also improving your poise and concentration. If standing is a challenge, this pose can be adapted to sitting, extending one leg out and pressing the sole of the foot to the inner thigh of the opposite leg, mimicking the standing version's posture.

Seated Eagle Pose

Another effective balance-focused pose is the seated eagle pose.

- While seated, wrap your one arm under the other, joining the palms if possible. This pose not only enhances your balance but also stretches the shoulders, upper back, and thighs. It's a compact pose that packs in a lot of benefits for both your body and mind, improving focus and stability.

- Hold for five to ten seconds and gradually increase the time as you progress.

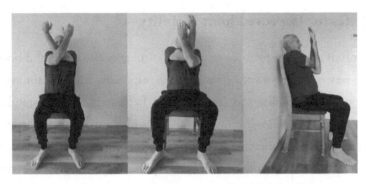

Breathing and relaxation techniques, or pranayama, are integral aspects of yoga. They help centre your mind, reduce stress, and improve your respiratory efficiency. One simple technique is the diaphragmatic breathing, where you focus on breathing deeply into your belly rather than your chest. This type of breathing encourages full oxygen exchange and is quite calming. Another technique is the alternate nostril breathing, which involves closing one nostril while breathing in, then closing the other while breathing out, and vice versa. This can help clear the mind and balance the body, making it a perfect practice to integrate into your daily routine, perhaps before bedtime or upon waking.

As you progress with these poses, it's important to listen to your body and understand how to safely increase their difficulty or adapt them to better suit your needs. This might mean holding a pose for longer periods, incorporating more challenging versions of the pose, or gradually reducing the reliance on the chair for support. Always prioritise safety and comfort, ensuring that the modifications you make serve to enhance your yoga practice without straining your body.

Yoga is not just a form of exercise; it's a tool for maintaining and enhancing your overall well-being. By incorporating these low-impact poses and breathing techniques into your life, you are taking steps not only to improve your physical health but also to enrich your mental and emotional landscape. So, embrace these gentle movements, breathe deeply, and enjoy the calm and strength that yoga brings into your life.

6.4 Pilates for Improved Joint Mobility

Pilates, often seen as a form of exercise that marries the mind and body, is a fantastic way to improve your overall fitness, especially if you're aiming to enhance your joint mobility and core strength. Let's start by understanding the core principles of Pilates—it centres on the idea of control rather than exertion. Unlike some forms of exercise that emphasise big, forceful movements, Pilates focuses on small, precise movements that require you to use your core muscles, the powerhouse of your body. This method not only helps in strengthening these muscles but also teaches you how to align your body correctly, which can reduce pain and increase mobility.

Diving into some beginner-friendly Pilates exercises.

Pelvic Curl

The pelvic curl is a great place to start. It's gentle yet extremely effective in activating the lower back, hips, and core.

- While lying flat on your back with your knees bent and feet flat on the floor, slowly peel your spine off the floor, starting from the tailbone and moving up vertebra by vertebra until your body forms a diagonal line from your shoulders to your knees.

- Hold for 15 – 30 seconds, repeat five times.

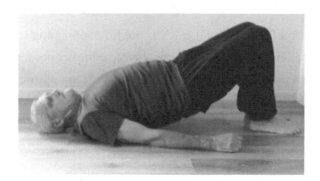

This exercise not only warms up the spine but also engages the deep abdominal muscles, enhancing both flexibility and strength.

Single Leg Curl

Another beneficial Pilates move is the single-leg circle.

- Lay on your back with one leg extended upwards and circling it gently. This works the hip joint and leg muscles, improving your range of motion and reducing stiffness.

- Do five to ten circles in each direction, then switch legs.

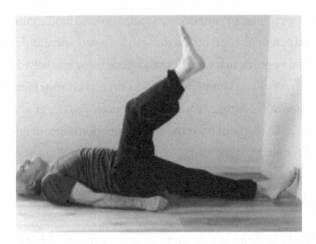

For those who might want to explore equipment-based Pilates, tools like the reformer or the magic circle offer a way to deepen your practice. The reformer, for instance, is a bed-like frame with a flat platform on it, called the carriage, which rolls back and forth on wheels within the frame. The resistance provided by the reformer's springs is what makes it so unique—it allows for a range of exercises that can be adjusted to different levels of difficulty. Using this equipment under the guidance of a trained professional can significantly enhance your strength, flexibility, and balance. The magic circle, a flexible ring that provides resistance, is another tool that can be used to perform exercises that target the muscles in the legs, arms, and trunk. These tools not only add variety to your workouts but also introduce a level of resistance that can be adjusted to suit your fitness level, making Pilates a very adaptable form of exercise.

Pilates is particularly effective in rehabilitation scenarios. Its focus on controlled, flowing motions and maintaining alignment makes it an excellent choice for those recovering from injuries or managing chronic conditions like arthritis. It helps increase joint mobility and decrease pain, which can significantly improve your quality of life. The adaptability of Pilates exercises means they can be customised to cater to your specific needs, focusing on areas that require rehabilitation. For instance, if you are recovering from a knee injury, specific Pilates exercises can be tailored to strengthen the muscles around the knee without placing undue stress on the joint.

Incorporating Pilates into your routine offers more than just physical benefits; it encourages an awareness of your body's capabilities and limitations, promoting a balanced approach to physical fitness that can keep you active and agile. Whether you're performing gentle mat exercises at home or using specialised equipment in a studio, Pilates provides a comprehensive way to enhance your joint mobility and core strength. As you continue with these practices, you might find a newfound appreciation for the way your body moves and functions, encouraging a healthier, more active lifestyle.

6.5 Using Resistance Bands for Strength Training

Let's talk about resistance bands, those stretchy strips of rubber that might just become your new favourite workout buddies. These bands are a fantastic tool for seniors because they're not just versatile and easy to use; they're also incredibly effective at building strength without putting undue stress on your joints. Think of resistance bands as your adjustable weight set. Depending on how you use them—whether you stretch them a little or a lot—you can control the intensity of your workout. This makes them ideal for a customised exercise session that fits exactly what your body needs on any given day.

Starting with some upper body exercises, resistance bands can be used to perform movements like band pull-apart or chest presses. These exercises are crucial because they target muscles that are vital for everyday activities. For band pull-apart, simply hold a resistance band with both hands in front of you, arms extended, and then pull the band apart by moving your arms to the sides. This exercise works the muscles in your upper back and shoulders, which helps in maintaining an upright posture—a key factor in good balance. Chest presses with a band can be done by anchoring the band behind you (you can use a closed door or a heavy piece of furniture) and pressing the ends of the band forward as if you were using a chest press machine at the gym. This strengthens your chest and arms, helping you with tasks that require pushing, like opening doors or stroller handling if you're spending time with your grandchildren.

Now, let's shift focus to the lower body, which is just as important for maintaining balance and stability. Resistance bands are excellent for exercises like seated leg presses or standing hip extensions. For a seated leg press, sit on a chair with a band looped around your feet, holding the ends with your hands. Press your feet forward against the band's resistance and then slowly return to the starting position. This mimics the leg press machine at gyms, targeting your thighs and glutes. For standing hip extensions, tie a band around your ankle and anchor it to a stable point behind you. Gently extend your leg backward against the band's resistance, working the glute muscles on that leg. These exercises not only increase the strength of your legs and hips but also improve your stability, making it easier to walk, climb stairs, or stand from a seated position.

Incorporating resistance bands into your daily routine can be both fun and effective. Think of creative ways to blend band exercises with your everyday activities. For instance, you can do a few stretches with the band while waiting for your morning coffee to brew or perform some seated exercises while watching your favourite TV show. Keeping a resistance band in your living room or kitchen is a great reminder to sneak in some exercise throughout the day. This not only keeps your muscles engaged but also ensures that your joints remain flexible, which is crucial for maintaining mobility as you age.

Resistance bands are not just tools for physical therapy; they are instruments of independence. They allow you to build strength safely and effectively, ensuring that your body remains capable of handling the demands of daily life. By incorporating these simple exercises into your routine, you're taking proactive steps to maintain your health and vitality, giving you the freedom to enjoy life on your terms.

Wrapping Up Strength Training and Looking Ahead

This chapter has taken you through various exercises using resistance bands, emphasising their role in building upper and lower body strength and incorporating them into your daily routines. These exercises are more than just movements; they are stepping stones to greater independence and confidence in your physical abilities. By consistently incorporating these resistance band exercises, you're not only working on your physical wellness but also ensuring that your daily life remains vibrant and active.

As we close this chapter on strength training and move forward, remember that each exercise and each day of practice brings you closer to a more balanced, stable, and fulfilling lifestyle. Up next, we'll explore lifestyle integration techniques that will help you blend all these exercises seamlessly into your everyday life, ensuring that your journey towards better balance and mobility continues to be as enjoyable and effective as possible. Stay tuned, and let's keep moving forward together!

Make a Difference with Your Review

Unlock the Power of Generosity

HEY THERE!

A few years ago, in my mid-sixties, I started to feel the effects of aging. Persistent aches and that non-physical exhaustion had become part of my daily life and a few falls from some balance issues I was having. While I kept up with regular walks, I realised something was missing. Then, something amazing happened—just half an hour of exercise per week transformed my life for the better.

Now, let's talk about you.

Would you lend a hand to someone you've never met, even if you'll never get credit for it? You may be wondering, "Who is this person?" Well, they might remind you of yourself—less experienced, eager to make a change, and needing guidance but not knowing where to find it.

That's why I created this book, and my mission is simple: to make *Balance Exercises for Seniors* accessible to everyone. Every book I write stems from that mission. And to achieve it, I need your help to reach...well...everyone.

Most people do judge a book by its cover—and its reviews. So here's my humble ask, not for me, but for a senior you've never met who's in need of support.

If you want to experience that 'feel-good' feeling and make a real difference, all it takes is a quick review. That's it.

If you're the kind of person who feels great about helping someone you don't know, then you're my kind of person. Welcome to the club—you're one of us!

And I can't wait to help you find relief, balance, and independence through the empowering exercises in this book.

From the bottom of my heart, thank you. Now, back to our regularly scheduled programming!

Your biggest fan,
Laurel Harris

Scan the QR code to leave your review!

CHAPTER 7

LIFESTYLE INTEGRATION

I MAGINE TURNING EVERYDAY CHORES into a fun balance-boosting routine! Whether you're washing dishes or sorting laundry, each mundane task hides a golden opportunity to enhance your stability and mobility. Think about it—why not make the most of the time you spend on chores by integrating some simple balance exercises? Not only does this help improve your balance, but it also makes these everyday tasks a bit more engaging.

7.1 Balance Exercises While Doing Household Chores

When it comes to household chores, there's more to them than meets the eye. These routine tasks are perfect moments to sneak in some balance training. For instance, while washing dishes at the sink, why not practice standing on one leg? It's simple: stand straight, lift one foot slightly off the ground, and hold that pose for as long as you can, then switch legs. This not only helps strengthen your leg muscles but also challenges your balance in a safe and controlled environment. Similarly, when folding laundry, you can intermittently perform toe-standing. Just rise up on your toes and hold for a few seconds before lowering back down. This exercise is excellent for activating the muscles in your calves and feet, which play crucial roles in maintaining balance.

Now, let's talk about moving safely while you're bustling around the house. It's essential to adopt safe movement patterns to prevent any falls and to train your body to move correctly. For example, when you need to pick something up from the floor, instead of bending over from the waist, try squatting. Keep your back straight and bend at your knees and hips, lowering yourself down as if you're going to sit on an imaginary chair. This method not only protects your back but also engages your leg muscles, similar to the mechanics of a squat exercise, which is excellent for strengthening and balance.

Furthermore, your home is filled with everyday items that can double as props for your balance exercises. Take your kitchen countertop, for example. While waiting for the kettle to boil or the microwave to ping, use the countertop for support and perform a series of calf raises—rise up on your toes and slowly lower back down. This not only helps build strength in your lower legs but also aids in improving your balance. Chairs can also be fantastic aids. Try standing behind a chair and practising mini leg lifts to the back and side to strengthen different muscle groups and enhance your overall stability.

Creating a Balanced Chore Routine

To make the most out of integrating balance exercises into your chores, it's wise to alternate between tasks that are more demanding on your balance and those that are less so. This approach helps prevent fatigue and keeps the routine manageable and enjoyable. Start with something simple, like wiping down the kitchen counter while on tiptoes, then move on to a more balance-intensive task like using a step stool to reach higher shelves. After that, switch back to a less demanding task. This way, you're not only keeping your body engaged but also giving it ample time to recover between more challenging activities.

By transforming household chores into opportunities for balance training, you not only make these everyday tasks more dynamic and enjoyable but also contribute significantly to your overall health and stability. This integration of balance exercises into daily routines is an effortless way to ensure you're consistently working on your mobility, making every day a step towards a stronger and more balanced you. So next time you're doing chores, remember, that every moment has the potential to be a balance-boosting opportunity. Embrace these activities with enthusiasm and watch as your stability and confidence soar, one chore at a time.

7.2 Incorporating Balance Work into Leisure Activities

When you think about leisure time, it's all about unwinding and enjoying activities that bring you joy and relaxation. But what if I told you that these leisurely moments could also double as an opportunity to enhance your balance and coordination? Engaging in activities you love, like gardening or dancing, can naturally incorporate balance work without feeling like a workout session. For instance, gardening is not just about planting flowers or vegetables; it involves various movements that challenge your balance. Reaching, bending, and squatting are all part of the gardening dance, and each one can be seen as a chance to strengthen your muscles and stability. Consider the act of reaching for a plant on the far side of a bed while maintaining your balance, or the squatting movement required to plant seeds. Each of these actions, performed mindfully, can significantly contribute to your balance training.

Dancing, particularly social forms like ballroom or line dancing, is another delightful way to enhance your balance. These dance forms require good coordination and control as you move in rhythm with a partner or group. The steps often involve quick changes in direction and pace, all of which naturally improve your dynamic balance and agility. What's more, the social aspect of dancing adds a wonderful, joyful element to the exercise, making it something to look forward to rather than a chore. Imagine gliding across the dance floor, the music lifting your spirits while each step also lifts your health and balance capabilities.

Turning our attention indoors, even watching TV can become an opportunity to sneak in some balance exercises. During commercial breaks, try standing behind your chair and performing leg lifts or standing marches. These simple activities keep your body active even during downtime and can significantly enhance your lower body strength and stability. Alternatively, while seated, you can perform ankle circles or flex and point your toes. These movements help keep your leg muscles engaged and improve circulation, contributing to better balance and reducing the risk of stiffness from sitting too long.

Lastly, consider hobbies that require dexterity and fine motor skills, such as knitting or model building. These activities might seem sedentary, but they actually help to enhance your cognitive function and hand-eye coordination, which are crucial for maintaining balance and stability. The precise movements involved in knitting, for example, not only improve finger dexterity but also keep your mind actively engaged, which is essential for overall brain health and balance control. Engaging regularly in such hobbies offers a dual benefit: keeping your mind sharp and your body in tune, all while doing something enjoyable.

By integrating balance activities into your leisure time, you transform routine or recreational activities into valuable moments of health and wellness enhancement. This approach ensures that maintaining balance and mobility becomes a seamless, enjoyable part of your everyday life, keeping you active, engaged, and happy in your pursuits. So next time you plan your leisure activities, think about how you can tweak them to include some balance work. It's a fun, rewarding way to enhance your stability and enjoy your favourite pastimes even more.

7.3 Using Technology to Enhance Routine and Track Progress

In the ever-evolving landscape of technology, there are innovative tools that can significantly enhance the way you approach balance training and overall fitness. Let's dive into the world of apps and wearable devices that are not just high-tech, but also incredibly user-friendly, designed to make your exercise routine more productive and enjoyable.

Starting with smartphone applications, there are numerous options available that can guide you through balance exercises with ease. These apps often come with detailed visual and auditory instructions to ensure you perform each movement safely and effectively. Picture an app that not only demonstrates the exercise but also provides real-time feedback on your posture and technique, just like a personal trainer would. For instance, some apps use the phone's camera to monitor your movements and give corrective advice, ensuring you get the most out of each session. Additionally, many of these applications include games that are designed to improve coordination and stability, making the process of balance training fun and engaging. Imagine playing a game where you need to tilt your phone to navigate a maze or balance a virtual object on the screen, all the while improving your physical skills.

Wearable technology, such as fitness trackers, takes this a step further by continuously monitoring your movements and providing insightful feedback on your activity levels throughout the day. These devices can be fantastic motivators. They track steps, measure how much you stand during the day, and remind you to keep moving if you've been inactive for too long. More advanced models can even analyse your walking pattern and suggest improvements to enhance your stability. It's like having a coach who's always with you, keeping an eye on your progress and pushing you towards your goals. Wearables can also track your heart rate, sleep patterns, and overall fitness levels, providing a comprehensive overview of your health that can be incredibly motivating.

The digital world also offers fantastic platforms for community interaction and support through online forums and social media groups dedicated to senior fitness. These communities are treasure troves of shared experiences, tips, and encouragement. You can connect with people who are on the same path, share your progress, ask for advice, or even join virtual challenges and activities. Sometimes, just knowing that others are out there with similar goals can be incredibly reassuring and motivating. You might read a post about someone who improved their balance and was able to go hiking again, or someone else who managed to reduce their fear of falling simply by adhering to a daily exercise routine shared in the group. These stories can inspire you to keep pushing forward, enhancing your commitment to your own balance goals.

Lastly, let's touch upon an exciting advancement in exercise technology: virtual reality (VR). VR systems can transport you to a completely controlled environment where you can practice balance exercises without any risk of falling. Imagine putting on a VR headset and finding yourself on a virtual beach, where you can walk along the shore, navigate around obstacles, or even play balance-enhancing games like virtual volleyball. The realistic scenarios not only make the exercises more enjoyable but also train your body and mind to handle similar situations in the real world. This kind of immersive experience is particularly beneficial for those who may be limited by space at home or who need a safe environment to practice challenging balance tasks.

By incorporating these technological tools into your balance training regimen, you open up a new world of possibilities that make staying active and improving your balance not just a goal, but an enjoyable part of your daily life. Whether through interactive apps, wearable devices, supportive online communities, or immersive VR experiences, technology offers you an array of exciting tools to enhance your routine, track your progress, and stay engaged in your quest for better balance and health. So why not take advantage of these modern solutions and make them a part of your journey towards a more stable and fulfilling lifestyle?

7.4 Community and Social Activities That Improve Balance

Imagine stepping out of your home and finding yourself in a vibrant community space where every activity you participate in not only boosts your balance but also connects you with friendly faces. This isn't just a pleasant daydream—it's a practical and enjoyable reality many seniors can tap into through various community and social activities.

Starting with group exercise classes, local community centres or gyms often offer programs specifically tailored to seniors. Picture yourself in a Tai Chi class where every slow, deliberate movement not only enhances your physical balance but also calms your mind. Or visualize participating in a gentle yoga session where you can stretch and strengthen your body in the company of others who share your goals and challenges. Water aerobics is another fantastic option that many find enjoyable. The buoyancy of the water makes it easier on your joints while the resistance helps build the muscle strength crucial for good balance. These classes often become more than just exercise sessions; they're a chance to meet new friends, share experiences, and support each other's progress. It's about creating a joyful routine that you look forward to, knowing you're not just improving your health but also enriching your social life.

Volunteering is another avenue that wonderfully blends physical activity with social engagement. Consider opportunities like helping out in a community garden. This isn't just about planting and weeding; it's about bending, stretching, and walking—all of which are great for your balance. It also connects you with nature and like-minded individuals, making it a deeply fulfilling activity that feeds your body, mind, and spirit. Additionally, participating in charity walks not only gets your legs moving but also brings a sense of accomplishment and community spirit. Each step you take isn't just a move towards better health—it's a stride towards helping others, which adds a beautiful layer of purpose to your physical activities.

Engaging in senior sports leagues offers another layer of fun and fitness. Sports such as bowling and golf require precision, control, and balance, making them perfect for gently challenging your stability. These activities also offer a fantastic way to indulge in some friendly competition and camaraderie. The social interactions involved can significantly enhance your mood and mental health, which are just as important as your physical well-being. Imagine the laughter and stories shared over a game of golf or the cheers in a bowling alley celebrating a strike. These moments build a sense of community and belonging, which is essential at any stage of life.

Lastly, don't overlook the value of attending community safety workshops. These events, often hosted by local health organisations or hospitals, are treasure troves of information. They provide practical tips on fall prevention and balance improvement, which are crucial for maintaining your independence. But more than just learning, these workshops are an opportunity to connect with professionals and peers who can offer support and advice tailored to your needs. It's about being proactive in your well-being and taking charge of your health in a supportive, community setting.

Each of these activities provides a dual benefit: they help improve your balance and physical health while also enriching your social life. Engaging in these community and social activities means you're never just working on your balance—you're building friendships, sharing experiences, and enjoying a vibrant social life, all of which contribute to a happier, healthier you. So, step out and explore the opportunities your community offers. It's a chance to live life more fully, supported by a network of friends and activities that keep you fit, active, and connected.

7.5 Balance and Mobility Tips for Travelling

Travelling can be one of life's greatest joys, offering new sights, sounds, and experiences. However, it can also present unique challenges, especially when it comes to maintaining balance and mobility. Preparing your body for the demands of travel can make your journey smoother and more enjoyable. Let's explore some effective ways to gear up for your next adventure.

Before you even pack your suitcase, consider starting a simple exercise routine that focuses on strengthening and stabilising the muscles you'll use most while travelling. For instance, if your vacation involves a lot of walking, prioritise leg and core strengthening exercises. Squats, leg lifts, and planks are fantastic for building the muscles in your lower body and core, providing you with a sturdier base and better balance. Additionally, practising balance-specific exercises like standing on one leg or heel-to-toe walking can be extremely beneficial. These exercises mimic the actions you'll likely perform on uneven cobblestone streets or while navigating through crowded airports. Just a few minutes each day leading up to your trip can significantly enhance your stability and endurance, making those long tour days less daunting.

Once you're on your way, finding time and space for exercise might seem tricky, but it's definitely manageable with a bit of creativity. Long flights or train rides can be tough on your body, especially if you're confined to a seat for extended periods. Use this time to engage in gentle seated exercises. Simple ankle rolls and foot pumps can improve circulation and prevent stiffness, while seated leg lifts and abdominal bracing can keep your core and legs active. If space allows, occasionally standing up and performing balance exercises like shifting weight from one foot to the other can also be beneficial. Similarly, when you're in your hotel room, a quick morning balance routine can energise you for the day's activities. Use the back of a chair or the edge of the bed for support while you do a series of mini squats or leg extensions.

Choosing the right footwear is crucial when travelling. The shoes you select can greatly impact your comfort and balance, especially when you're exploring new places. Look for shoes with good arch support, non-slip soles, and enough cushioning to absorb shocks from walking on hard surfaces. Proper footwear not only prevents fatigue but also reduces the risk of slips, trips, and falls, ensuring you can wander worry-free. Make sure to break in new shoes before your trip to avoid blisters or discomfort, and always pack an extra pair just in case one gets wet or uncomfortable.

For those who find maintaining balance particularly challenging, or if you're travelling to destinations with uneven terrain, consider using mobility aids. Walking sticks or trekking poles can be invaluable tools. They not only provide an extra point of contact with the ground but also distribute your weight more evenly, which can alleviate pressure on your knees and hips. This is particularly helpful when climbing hills or navigating slippery pathways. Most are lightweight and collapsible, making them easy to pack and carry. Don't view these aids as a sign of limitation but rather as tools that enable you to explore more freely and safely.

By incorporating these strategies into your travel plans, you ensure that mobility and balance issues don't hold you back from enjoying your adventures to the fullest. With a bit of preparation, the right exercises, and the appropriate gear, you can embrace the joys of travel with confidence and ease.

As we wrap up this chapter, remember, that every tip and exercise shared here is a stepping stone towards more confident and enjoyable travels. Whether you're exploring the ancient ruins of Rome or the vibrant streets of Tokyo, maintaining your balance and mobility enhances your experience, allowing you to soak in every moment without worry. This chapter not only prepares you for the journeys you'll embark on but also ensures that each trip is as rewarding as possible. As we move forward, let's carry this spirit of preparedness and adaptability into all areas of life, ensuring that no matter where we are, we're always ready to step confidently and enjoy every experience life has to offer.

CHAPTER 8

OVERCOMING CHALLENGES AND SETBACKS

I MAGINE YOU'RE ON A leisurely stroll through your favourite park, but un-expectedly, the path gets a bit rocky. The scenery is still breathtaking, but the walk becomes a bit more challenging. Much like this walk, your journey to better balance might encounter some rough patches. It's all part of the adventure, and while these setbacks might seem like obstacles, they're actually opportunities to grow stronger and more resilient. This chapter is dedicated to helping you navigate these moments with grace and determination.

8.1 Addressing Setbacks and How to Stay Motivated

Understanding Setbacks as Part of the Process

First things first, let's redefine setbacks. Instead of viewing them as failures, think of them as integral parts of the learning curve—each one offers a unique insight into your progress and process. It's normal to have days where exercises seem harder, or your balance feels off. These moments don't define your journey; they refine it. Recognising that setbacks are not stop signs but part of the normal ebb and flow can transform your approach, turning frustration into a moment of learning. What can each setback teach you? Maybe it's telling you to slow down, focus more on form, or even that it's time to take a well-deserved rest.

Strategies for Overcoming Discouragement

When discouragement knocks on your door, having a toolkit ready can help you stay the course. Start by setting smaller, achievable goals. If balancing for 30 seconds feels overwhelming, scale it back to 15 seconds and gradually increase your time. Celebrate when you meet these smaller targets—it's about progress, not perfection. Consistency is another powerful tool. Try to incorporate your balance exercises into your daily routine, making them as habitual as your morning cup of coffee. Adjusting expectations is crucial too. Progress isn't always linear; some days will feel like a breeze, and others like a climb. Adjust your expectations to embrace this variability, which in itself can be a motivator to keep pushing forward.

Maintaining a Positive Mindset

The power of positive thinking isn't just a cliché; it's a fundamental part of overcoming setbacks. Cultivate a mindset that embraces challenges and views them as opportunities for growth. Techniques like affirmations can be incredibly powerful. Start your day by affirming your abilities: "I am improving my balance every day." Mindfulness meditation can also help centre your thoughts and reduce stress, making you less likely to be swayed by temporary setbacks. Practising mindfulness can involve simply spending a few minutes each day in quiet reflection, focusing on your breath and the sensations in your body. This practice not only calms the mind but also deeply connects you with the physical body and its capabilities.

Inspirational Stories of Overcoming Challenges

Sometimes, hearing about others who have walked a similar path and faced similar challenges can light a spark of motivation. Consider the story of Michael, a 76-year-old who started balance exercises after a minor fall that shook his confidence. Initially, Michael felt disheartened by his slow progress and occasional setbacks. However, by setting small, daily goals and celebrating each achievement, he slowly saw improvements. Within months, not only did his balance improve, but his confidence soared. Michael's story isn't just about improving balance; it's about reclaiming independence and joy in everyday activities. Let such stories remind you that the road might be bumpy, but the destination of improved balance and enhanced life quality is well within reach.

Through understanding and embracing setbacks, employing strategies to combat discouragement, maintaining a positive outlook, and drawing inspiration from others' journeys, you can navigate the ups and downs of improving your balance. Remember, each step, no matter how small, is a step forward. Keep moving, keep adjusting, and keep your eyes on the path ahead, filled with opportunities and new horizons.

8.2 Modifying Exercises for Fluctuating Health Issues

Navigating through life with fluctuating health issues, such as arthritis, back pain, or temporary injuries, can feel like trying to dance on a moving carpet. It's unpredictable, and what worked yesterday might not feel right today. This is why adapting your exercise routine to accommodate these changes isn't just helpful—it's essential. Adaptive exercise techniques can be life-changing, providing you with flexibility and control over your workout, ensuring you continue to benefit without exacerbating your condition.

Let's talk about arthritis, for instance. This condition can make movements painful and challenging, but that doesn't mean you should stop moving altogether. In fact, keeping your joints active is crucial. Modifying exercises to make them arthritis-friendly means focusing on low-impact movements that don't strain your joints. For example, if a standard squat is too painful, a seated version where you rise from a chair to a standing position and back down can be just as effective at strengthening your legs and core without stressing your knees. Similarly, for back pain, exercises that strengthen your core and alleviate pressure on the spine can be incorporated into your routine. Techniques like pelvic tilts or gentle stretches performed in a warm pool can reduce discomfort and improve mobility.

Now, let's consider the invaluable advice you can receive from healthcare providers. Regular consultations with your doctor or physical therapist are vital, especially when your health conditions change. They can provide guidance on which exercises are safe and beneficial, and which should be avoided. They can also show you how to correctly perform each exercise to maximise benefits and minimise risk. For example, a physical therapist might demonstrate how to use a resistance band to improve your shoulder mobility without exacerbating existing pain, or they may recommend specific stretches to alleviate sciatica symptoms.

Implementing assistive devices into your exercise routine can also make a significant difference in your safety and effectiveness. Tools like walking aids or braces stabilise your movements and can boost your confidence immensely. For instance, using a walking stick can help you maintain your balance during outdoor walks, reducing the fear of falling. Braces, on the other hand, provide support to weakened joints or muscles, allowing you to perform exercises with better form. Supportive footwear is another game-changer, specially designed to provide extra cushion and support, they can help in evenly distributing your body weight, taking the stress off painful joints.

Flexibility in your exercise routine is another key element. It's important to listen to your body and understand that it's okay to modify your activities based on how you feel each day. If you wake up feeling stiff and sore, it might be a day for gentle stretching rather than more vigorous balance exercises. Or, if you're experiencing an arthritis flare-up, switching to water aerobics where the buoyancy of the water helps reduce joint stress can be a wise move. The goal is to maintain activity without pushing your body into discomfort or pain.

By embracing adaptive exercise techniques, consulting healthcare professionals for personalised advice, using assistive devices, and maintaining flexibility in your routine, you can continue to enjoy the benefits of exercise in a way that respects and responds to your body's needs. This approach not only helps in managing your symptoms but also empowers you to take charge of your health and well-being, ensuring that your exercise routine is a source of strength and joy, rather than discomfort or dread. Remember, each modification is a step towards maintaining your mobility and independence, making your workout routine a true ally in your health journey.

8.3 Coping with the Fear of Falling

Imagine for a moment that the simple act of walking across a room didn't just involve the physical steps, but also carried a shadow of fear with each move. For many seniors, this isn't just a thought experiment—it's daily life. The fear of falling is profound and real, but it doesn't have to define your life. There are empowering and effective strategies that can not only reduce this fear but also equip you with the confidence to move freely and safely.

One of the most effective ways to tackle this fear is through educational workshops on fall prevention. These sessions are more than just informative—they're transformative. They provide practical tips and techniques on how to navigate your environment safely, make adjustments to your home to minimise fall risks, and exercises that enhances balance and strength. Community centres, local hospitals, or senior centres often host these workshops. They serve as a great opportunity to learn in a supportive group setting, where you can also share experiences and tips with peers who understand what you're going through. Knowledge is power, and understanding the mechanics of falling and how to prevent it can significantly lessen your fear.

Practical strategies also play a crucial role in managing the fear of falling. Simple practices like learning the correct way to fall can reduce the risk of serious injury. It sounds counterintuitive—learning to fall? But it's similar to the techniques taught in martial arts, such as tucking your chin and rolling with the fall, which distribute the impact more broadly across your body. Practising getting up safely from a fall is equally important. Use a sturdy piece of furniture to steady yourself and practice rising in a controlled manner. These are invaluable skills that give you confidence in your ability to handle a fall, should it ever happen.

Building confidence through mastery of balance exercises is another cornerstone of overcoming the fear of falling. Start with simple exercises, gradually increasing their difficulty as your confidence grows. This could be something as simple as standing on one foot while holding onto a chair, and gradually progressing to doing it without support. Each small victory in these exercises builds not just physical strength, but mental assurance too. Celebrate these milestones, no matter how small they may seem. Mastery of these exercises translates into a broader sense of control and autonomy, reducing the fear associated with falling.

For some, the fear of falling might feel overwhelming, seeping into various aspects of life and preventing even basic activities. In such cases, therapeutic approaches like cognitive-behavioural therapy (CBT) can be incredibly beneficial. CBT helps in identifying and changing negative thought patterns that contribute to the fear of falling. It teaches coping mechanisms and ways to gradually face and overcome these fears in a controlled and safe manner. Counselling sessions can also provide a safe space to discuss fears and anxieties, often uncovering underlying issues that might be contributing to the fear. These professional therapies can guide you through emotional hurdles, restoring your confidence and peace of mind.

Dealing with the fear of falling isn't just about preventing falls; it's about enriching your quality of life, and ensuring that fear doesn't keep you from enjoying your golden years. By educating yourself, adopting practical safety measures, mastering balance-enhancing exercises, and seeking professional help when needed, you can navigate this challenge effectively. Remember, every step taken to combat this fear is a step toward a more confident and active life. Embrace these strategies, and let them guide you to a path where mobility is met with confidence, not fear.

8.4 Engaging Family and Friends for Support and Motivation

Imagine your balance training not just as a solo endeavour but as a communal dance, involving those closest to you—your family and friends. Their role in your fitness journey can be profoundly impactful, transforming the experience from a routine task into a shared joy. Creating a support network of loved ones who understand and actively support your goals can significantly enhance your motivation and commitment. It's about building a circle of encouragement, where each member uplifts and inspires the others.

Think about it—having someone by your side, cheering you on, can make a world of difference. This network might include your spouse, children, close friends, or even neighbours. They can provide not just emotional support, but also practical help. Perhaps it's your daughter reminding you gently about your afternoon exercises, or a neighbour who joins you for a balance-focused yoga session. Each act of support, big or small, reinforces your commitment to maintaining and improving your balance.

Involving your loved ones in your exercises can also be a wonderful way to spend quality time together. You could introduce a weekly session where family members or friends join you in your balance routine, or perhaps they could accompany you to a Tai Chi class in the park. These shared activities not only help you stick to your exercise regimen but also enhance the enjoyment of the process. It's about making these moments fun and engaging, turning them into opportunities for laughter and bonding. For instance, you could have a balance challenge with your grandchildren, seeing who can stand on one leg the longest, turning it into a game that everyone looks forward to.

Setting shared fitness goals with friends or family can also be incredibly motivating. When you commit to a goal with someone else, it creates a sense of accountability that can drive you to stick with your routine, especially on days when motivation is low. These goals don't have to be huge; they could be as simple as "We'll both do our balance exercises at least four times a week," or "We'll attend three yoga classes this month." Celebrating these achievements together can be very rewarding. Perhaps you could set a joint reward for meeting your goals, like treating yourselves to a concert or a special meal.

Celebrating successes together is crucial. Each milestone, whether it's improving your balance time by a few seconds or mastering a new yoga pose, deserves recognition. Organising small celebrations or outings to mark these achievements can significantly boost morale. It could be as simple as a special dinner at your favourite restaurant or a family gathering where everyone shares what they've accomplished. These celebrations not only acknowledge your hard work but also strengthen your connections with those around you, reinforcing the supportive framework that helps sustain your balance journey.

By weaving your balance exercises into the fabric of your relationships, you transform your pursuit of better stability into a collective adventure, enriched with support, laughter, and shared accomplishments. This approach not only makes the journey more enjoyable but also embeds your fitness goals into your social interactions, creating a robust support system that motivates and sustains you as you improve your balance and enhance your life.

8.5 Celebrating Milestones and Recognising Improvement

Setting milestones in your balance exercise routine isn't just about marking progress—it's about building a roadmap that guides and motivates you on your path to better stability. Think of milestones as lighthouses shining along a coastal drive; they reassure you that you're on the right track and encourage you to keep going. Start by setting realistic, achievable goals that reflect your current abilities and push you just enough to keep things challenging. For instance, if you're just starting out, a good milestone might be to balance on one foot for 10 seconds. As you improve, you could extend this time or add more complex exercises to your routine.

Keeping track of these milestones is crucial, and there are several tools at your disposal to help with this. Journals are fantastic for recording your daily exercises and any observations you have about your performance and how you feel. Digital apps offer another great way to monitor your progress, with features that allow you to set reminders, track your consistency, and sometimes even provide feedback on your form. Progress charts, either on paper or online, can offer a visual representation of your improvements over time, which can be incredibly satisfying and motivating to look at.

Recognising and celebrating every win along your exercise journey, no matter how small, is fundamental. These small victories, like increasing your balancing time by a few seconds or successfully completing a new exercise without support, are proof of your hard work and dedication. Celebrating these achievements can significantly boost your morale and motivation. It could be as simple as acknowledging your success at the end of your routine or rewarding yourself with something enjoyable, like a favourite treat or a relaxing bath. It's these moments of recognition that reinforce your commitment to your exercise regimen and make the process enjoyable.

Incorporating reflective practices into your routine can further enhance your appreciation of your journey. Journaling is a particularly effective method, allowing you to reflect on your daily exercises, the challenges you faced, and how you overcame them. This can be a profound source of personal insight and growth, helping you understand more about your body's capabilities and needs. Group discussions, whether in fitness classes or online forums, can also be invaluable. Sharing your experiences with others who are on similar paths not only fosters a sense of community but also provides diverse insights and encouragement that can bolster your own resolve and perhaps give you new ideas to improve your routine.

Creating personal reward systems can also play a crucial role in your exercise regimen. Setting up specific rewards for achieving your milestones can serve as powerful motivation. For instance, you might decide that once you've successfully balanced for 30 seconds, you'll attend a special event, or perhaps buy that book you've been eyeing. These rewards provide something tangible to strive for, making the goals more compelling and the journey towards them more exciting.

Adopting these practices—setting and tracking milestones, recognising and celebrating small wins, engaging in reflective practices, and establishing a reward system—transforms your approach to balance exercises from a daily task to a dynamic and rewarding part of your life. Each step you take is a step towards greater confidence and independence, and recognizing your progress only serves to push you further towards your goals.

As we wrap up this discussion on celebrating milestones and recognising improvement, remember that each small step forward is a significant achievement in your broader quest for better balance and health. These practices not only enhance your physical fitness but also enrich your mental and emotional well-being, making the journey as rewarding as the destination. Now, as we move forward, let's continue to build on this foundation, exploring holistic approaches to balance that integrate physical, mental, and nutritional strategies to support your overall stability and wellness.

CHAPTER 9

HOLISTIC APPROACHES TO BALANCE

As you've been working through these exercises, improving your balance and enhancing your mobility, have you ever wondered about the role your diet plays in all this? Sure, we often hear that "you are what you eat," but this goes beyond just managing your weight or keeping your heart healthy. The right nutrients can bolster your bones, aid your muscles, and even speed up recovery times, making a balanced diet an essential component of your balance training regimen. Let's dive into the world of nutrition and discover how the food you eat directly impacts your ability to stand firm and steady.

9.1 Nutrition Tips to Support Bone Health and Balance

Essential Nutrients for Bone Strength

When we talk about bone health, calcium often steals the spotlight, and rightly so. This mineral is the cornerstone of strong bones. Dairy products like milk, cheese, and yogurt are packed with calcium, but if you're not a fan of dairy, don't worry. You have plenty of other options like kale, broccoli, and almonds. But calcium doesn't work alone; it's part of a team that includes vitamin D, which helps your body absorb calcium effectively. While basking in the sun for a bit can boost your vitamin D levels, foods like fatty fish, egg yolks, and fortified foods also contribute to your intake.

Let's not forget about magnesium and potassium—these minerals also play crucial roles in bone health. Magnesium helps activate vitamin D, and without it, all the calcium and vitamin D intake might not be as effective. You can find magnesium in foods like whole grains, nuts, and green leafy vegetables. Potassium, on the other hand, helps neutralize acids that remove calcium from the body. Bananas, oranges, and potatoes are excellent sources of potassium. Integrating these nutrients into your daily diet can create a strong foundation, quite literally, by strengthening your bones and reducing your risk of falls.

Balanced Diet for Overall Health

A well-rounded diet is like a symphony where each nutrient plays its part in harmony, contributing to your overall health and balance. Protein strengthens muscles, which are crucial for good balance. Carbohydrates provide energy, which fuels all your activities, including those balance exercises. Fats are essential too; they're not just energy stores but are also vital for nerve health. And let's not overlook fibre, which keeps your digestive system running smoothly, ensuring that all these nutrients are efficiently absorbed.

Incorporating a variety of foods ensures that you get a broad spectrum of nutrients to support your balance training. Think colourful plates—fruits and vegetables of different colours provide different nutrients. Add lean proteins, whole grains, and healthy fats to round off your meals. This diversity not only nourishes your body but also makes your meals more enjoyable. After all, who doesn't love a vibrant, tasty dish that's also a feast for the eyes?

Supplementation Considerations

Sometimes, despite our best efforts, we might not get enough nutrients from our diet alone. This is where supplements can play a helpful role. For instance, if you're not getting enough sunlight, especially in the winter months, a vitamin D supplement might be necessary. However, it's crucial to approach supplements with caution and consult with a healthcare provider before starting any new supplement regimen. They can help you determine which supplements are necessary based on your specific needs and ensure that they won't interfere with any medications you're taking.

Impact of Nutrition on Recovery

Nutrition also plays a pivotal role in recovery, whether from everyday fatigue or more significant injuries. Proteins help repair muscle tissue, while vitamins and minerals like vitamin C and zinc support the immune system and speed up healing. Antioxidant-rich foods, such as berries and nuts, can help reduce inflammation, aiding in recovery and keeping you ready for your next balance session.

Eating well is about more than just satisfying hunger—it's about fueling and repairing your body, making it strong and resilient. Whether you're recovering from a slip or preparing for your next balance workout, the right nutrients can make all the difference. So, take a moment to reflect on your diet, and consider how you can adjust it to better support your balance and your overall health. Remember, every meal is an opportunity to enhance your stability, one bite at a time.

9.2 Mental Exercises to Enhance Focus and Mental Clarity

Just as you've been nurturing your body with balance exercises, it's equally important to keep your mind sharp and agile. Engaging in mental exercises can significantly enhance your cognitive functions, which, believe it or not, play a huge role in maintaining physical balance and stability. Let's explore some engaging activities that not only keep your mind active but also support your overall balance training efforts.

First off, consider the fun world of puzzles and memory games. These aren't just entertaining ways to pass the time; they're crucial tools for cognitive stimulation. Engaging regularly in crossword puzzles, Sudoku, or memory-matching games challenges your brain, improving both your short-term memory and problem-solving skills. These activities require you to think critically and make quick decisions, which can help enhance your mental agility. Over time, this can translate into quicker reflexes and better balance, as a sharp mind can better coordinate with your body's movements. If puzzles aren't your thing, how about learning something new? Taking up a new hobby, such as painting, learning a musical instrument, or even a new language, can stimulate neural pathways and keep your brain vibrant and engaged.

Shifting gears to meditation and mindfulness practices, these are not just trendy concepts but are proven techniques to enhance mental clarity and reduce stress. Regular practice of meditation can lead to significant improvements in your focus and attention to detail—key components in maintaining physical balance. When you meditate, you train your brain to focus on the present moment and clear out cluttering thoughts, which can help you stay centred both mentally and physically during balance exercises. Mindfulness, meanwhile, involves being acutely aware of what you're feeling and sensing at the moment, without interpretation or judgment. By practising mindfulness during your routine activities, you can enhance your sensory perceptions, which are crucial for maintaining stability and preventing falls.

The connection between mental and physical health is well-documented in research. Studies have shown that individuals who engage in regular mental and physical exercises tend to have better motor coordination and balance. This is particularly important as you age, as maintaining cognitive function plays a significant role in your overall ability to perform daily tasks independently. Regular mental training ensures that your brain remains capable of effectively communicating with your muscles, ensuring that your movements are more coordinated and balanced. It's all about creating a robust network between your mind and body, making sure each supports the other in maintaining your health and independence.

Now, how do you incorporate these mental exercises into your daily routine? It's simpler than you might think. Set aside a specific time each day for these activities, much like you would for physical exercises. Perhaps start your morning with a crossword puzzle or spend a few minutes meditating before breakfast. If you enjoy technology, there are numerous apps designed to improve cognitive function through fun and engaging games. Make it a part of your daily routine, just like a meal or a medication schedule. Consistency is key, and over time, these mental exercises will become as natural as your physical balance routines, enhancing both your mental acuity and your physical stability.

9.3 The Role of Hydration in Muscle Function and Balance

Staying sufficiently hydrated might not be the first thing you think about when it comes to maintaining your balance, but it plays a pivotal role in keeping your muscles functioning optimally. Just like oil in a machine, water helps ensure that your muscles work smoothly and efficiently. When your body is well-hydrated, your muscles are more elastic and less prone to stiffness, which can significantly affect your balance and coordination. Every muscle contraction and relaxation requires fluids to facilitate these movements—if your hydration levels are off, you might find your muscles reacting slower than usual or cramping up, both of which can throw off your balance and increase your risk of falls.

Cramps are more than just a painful nuisance; they are a direct signal from your body that it's lacking enough fluids to keep muscle cells working correctly. These spasms can be quite sudden and severe, causing your muscles to seize up when you least expect it. This is particularly risky when you're engaged in activities that require precise balance. Ensuring you drink enough water helps maintain the right balance of electrolytes in your muscles, preventing these cramps and keeping your movements smooth and coordinated.

Let's talk about how much water you should be drinking. While the old adage of eight glasses a day is a decent general guideline, the right amount can actually vary quite a bit depending on factors like your age, weight, and level of physical activity. As we age, our body's ability to conserve water decreases and our sense of thirst may not be as sharp, which can quickly lead us to drink less than we need. A good rule of thumb is to aim for about 1 to 1.5 millilitres of water per calorie consumed each day. For a typical senior consuming about 2000 calories a day, this translates to about 2 to 3 litres of water. However, if you're active and exercise regularly, you might need more to compensate for the fluid lost through sweat.

Monitoring your hydration status is crucial, and fortunately, your body gives you several signals to help you know if you're not drinking enough. Early signs of dehydration include feeling thirsty, dry mouth, and darker urine. As dehydration progresses, you might feel dizzy or confused—symptoms that directly impact your balance and overall safety. Maintaining an awareness of these signs can help you take action early, preventing the more severe effects of dehydration.

Increasing your fluid intake can sometimes feel like a chore, but there are several ways to make it more enjoyable and effective. Setting regular reminders on your phone or clock can help keep you on track until drinking water becomes a more natural part of your routine. If plain water doesn't excite your taste buds, try infusing it with natural flavours like slices of lemon, cucumber, or mint. These not only enhance the taste without adding sugar but can also make the idea of reaching for a glass more appealing. Furthermore, eating foods high in water content—such as cucumbers, tomatoes, oranges, and melons—can also contribute to your hydration levels, offering a nutritious bonus along with hydration.

Remember, keeping hydrated is more than just quenching your thirst; it's about providing your body with the essential elements it needs to maintain muscle function, flexibility, and balance. So, keep that water bottle handy and enjoy the refreshing path to maintaining your stability and health.

9.4 Relaxation Techniques to Reduce Stress and Improve Sleep

Reducing stress in your life is like giving a well-deserved break to your body and mind. It's not just about feeling better emotionally; stress reduction has tangible benefits for your physical health, particularly when it comes to maintaining balance and stability. When you're stressed, your body is in a constant state of alertness, which can make your muscles tense and your movements less coordinated. This tension not only makes it harder to maintain your balance but can also lead to fatigue, which further impacts your stability. By managing stress effectively, you can keep your muscles relaxed and your mind focused, both of which are essential for good balance.

Relaxation techniques are your tools for combating stress, and there are several effective methods you can easily integrate into your daily routine. Progressive muscle relaxation, for instance, involves tensing and then relaxing different muscle groups in your body. This technique not only helps alleviate muscle tension but also promotes a general sense of physical and mental relaxation. Here's how you can practice it: start with your feet and gradually work your way up to your face, tensing each muscle group for about five seconds and then slowly releasing the tension. As you release each muscle, imagine the stress flowing out of your body, leaving you calm and relaxed.

Deep breathing exercises are another cornerstone of stress management. By focusing on deep, slow breaths, you can activate your body's natural relaxation response. This not only helps reduce stress but also improves your focus, which is crucial for maintaining balance. Try this simple deep breathing exercise: sit comfortably with your back straight, and breathe in slowly through your nose, allowing your chest and lower belly to rise as you fill your lungs. Hold your breath briefly, then exhale slowly through your mouth or nose, whichever feels more comfortable. Repeating this process several times can help calm your mind and reduce muscle tension.

Guided imagery, or visualisation, is a powerful relaxation technique that involves imagining a scene in which you feel at peace, free to let go of all tension and anxiety. This could be a quiet beach, a serene garden, or any place that you find calming. Close your eyes and take a few deep breaths, then picture yourself in your peaceful place. Try to use all your senses to make the scene as vivid as possible—the sound of the waves, the smell of the saltwater, and the warmth of the sun on your skin. Spending a few minutes in your tranquil refuge can help reduce stress and improve your emotional and physical well-being.

Improving the quality of your sleep is another crucial aspect of reducing stress and enhancing your balance. Good sleep not only helps your body recover from the day's activities but also ensures that your nervous system functions optimally, keeping your mind clear and your movements coordinated. Establishing a soothing bedtime routine can significantly improve your sleep quality. This might include activities like reading a book, listening to soft music, or doing some gentle stretches—anything that signals to your body that it's time to wind down. Creating an ideal sleeping environment is also important; ensure your bedroom is quiet, dark, and cool, and invest in a comfortable mattress and pillows.

Integrating these relaxation techniques into your daily life can be as routine as your morning cup of coffee. Set aside specific times each day for these practices, just as you would for physical exercises. Whether it's starting your day with deep breathing, taking a midday break for some guided imagery, or unwinding with progressive muscle relaxation before bed, regular practice can enhance its effectiveness in reducing stress and improving your sleep. Over time, these practices not only contribute to better physical balance but also to a more joyful and fulfilling life.

9.5 The Importance of Regular Health Check-Ups

Keeping in touch with your healthcare providers isn't just about addressing illnesses when they arise; it's a proactive approach to maintaining your overall wellness and balance. Think of these regular check-ups as routine maintenance for your body, similar to servicing your car to keep it running smoothly. During these visits, your doctor can monitor any changes in your health that might affect your balance, such as alterations in your vision, hearing, or joint health. For instance, even slight changes in your hearing can impact your balance, as your ears play a critical role in helping you navigate space. Similarly, worsening vision can make it harder to see obstacles that might trip you up, and joint issues can make movements stiff and painful, affecting how well you can manage your balance.

The beauty of preventative care is that it helps catch potential health issues before they develop into more serious problems. Regular screenings for bone density can help detect osteoporosis early on, allowing you to take steps to strengthen your bones before you're at high risk of falls. Blood pressure and cholesterol levels can also impact your balance and overall health; monitoring these can help you make dietary or lifestyle changes that can improve both your health and your stability. It's all about catching things early and managing them effectively, ensuring that small issues don't turn into larger ones that could significantly impact your life and independence.

Medication reviews are another critical aspect of these check-ups. As we age, it's not uncommon to be on multiple medications, and each one comes with its own set of potential side effects. Some medications might cause dizziness, and drowsiness, or even affect your cognitive functions, all of which can severely impact your balance. Regularly reviewing these medications with your healthcare provider ensures that you are taking the right doses and that they're not interacting in ways that could be detrimental to your health or balance. It's also an opportunity to discuss any new symptoms or concerns you might have about your medications, allowing your doctor to make necessary adjustments.

Building a solid relationship with your healthcare providers can transform the way you manage your health. This isn't about just showing up to your appointments; it's about engaging actively with your doctors and health professionals. Be open about your lifestyle, your diet, your exercise habits, and any challenges you're facing. The more they know about your day-to-day life, the better they can tailor their advice and treatment plans to suit your needs. This collaborative approach ensures that every aspect of your health is being cared for, from your physical balance to your nutritional needs and your mental well-being.

By maintaining regular check-ups and a proactive relationship with your healthcare providers, you're not just looking after your health; you're ensuring that you remain active, independent, and balanced. So, make those appointments, and approach each visit as an opportunity to enhance your quality of life. It's your health, and taking control of it is a powerful step toward maintaining your balance and your independence.

Connecting to the Bigger Picture

Reflecting on this chapter, it's clear that balance is about more than just physical stability. It's a comprehensive blend of good nutrition, mental sharpness, proper hydration, stress management, and regular medical oversight. Each element is crucial in maintaining not only your physical balance but also your overall health and quality of life. As we move forward, remember that each aspect of your health is interconnected, and nurturing each one is key to staying balanced and vibrant.

In the next chapter, we'll explore how to maintain and build upon the balance skills you've developed, ensuring that you continue to enjoy a stable, active, and fulfilling life. Let's keep this momentum going, embracing each new day with confidence and vitality.

Chapter 10

Long-Term Balance Maintenance

I MAGINE YOUR DAILY ROUTINE as a garden. Just as a garden thrives with regular care—watering, weeding, and sun—so does your balance when nurtured daily with exercises and activities. It's about making small, sustainable habits that grow over time, helping you maintain your stability and mobility well into the future. This isn't just about adding years to your life, but life to your years, ensuring you can continue to do the things you love with confidence and independence.

10.1 Daily Routines for Sustained Balance and Mobility

Establishing Consistent Practice

Consistency is the golden thread that ties your balance exercises together into a strong, supportive tapestry. It's about weaving these practices into the fabric of your daily life so that they become as habitual as your morning cup of coffee. To build this consistency, it's helpful to anchor your balance exercises to specific times of the day. Maybe you start your morning by stretching before you even get out of bed, or perhaps you do a few balance stands while waiting for your lunch to cook. The evening might find you winding down with some gentle Tai Chi. By attaching exercises to regular daily activities, you set triggers that remind you to complete them, making it easier to build a routine that sticks.

Integration into Daily Activities

Let's get creative with how we can blend balance exercises into your everyday activities. For instance, while brushing your teeth, you can stand on one leg to challenge your stability—a simple yet effective way to enhance balance. Or, while waiting for the kettle to boil, why not perform a few heel raises? Turn hallway walks into an opportunity for heel-to-toe walking, transforming a simple transit from one room to another into a beneficial balance exercise. These integrations not only improve your balance but also break up the monotony of daily chores, adding an element of fun and challenge to ordinary routines.

Creating a Balanced Life

A truly balanced life extends beyond physical exercises; it encompasses social interactions and mental stimulation, which are just as crucial for your overall well-being. Engaging with friends and family, partaking in hobbies that challenge your mind and body, and even adopting pets can all contribute to a balanced lifestyle. These activities keep your mind sharp, your body active, and your spirit lifted. They also provide opportunities for laughter, love, and joy, which bolster your emotional health and, in turn, improve physical stability. After all, a happy, socially connected life is a cornerstone of holistic health.

Technology Aids

In our modern world, technology offers wonderful tools to help keep your balance exercises on track. Apps that you can download onto your smartphone can remind you to do your daily exercises and even guide you through various routines. Wearable devices like fitness trackers monitor your daily activity levels and provide feedback on your progress. Some can even detect stability and gait patterns, offering insights into your balance proficiency. These technological aids are not just gadgets; they are companions in your journey toward maintaining long-term balance and mobility, providing both reminders and encouragement right at your fingertips.

By setting a routine, integrating small exercises into your daily life, embracing a lifestyle that supports overall well-being, and utilising technology, you create a comprehensive approach to maintaining balance. This isn't just about preventing falls; it's about enhancing your ability to lead a full, active life. So, let's keep moving, keep balancing, and keep enjoying every step of this wonderfully balanced life you're cultivating.

10.2 Adapting Your Exercises as You Age Further

Life is a dance that changes its rhythm over time, and just as you adjust your steps to a new beat, so too should your approach to balance exercises evolve as you age. It's vital to reevaluate your physical abilities periodically. This doesn't just mean acknowledging limitations but also recognising and celebrating newfound strengths. Think of it like a regular tune-up for your car—it ensures everything runs smoothly, helping you avoid breakdowns. You might find that exercises that were once challenging are now comfortable, or perhaps some movements are not as easy as they used to be. This understanding allows you to adapt your routine, ensuring it remains aligned with your body's needs.

Modifying your exercise techniques plays a crucial role in maintaining safety and effectiveness. As we age, our joints and muscles might not be as forgiving, and high-impact exercises can become less feasible. This is where the beauty of adaptation comes in. For instance, if you've been doing standing balance exercises that now feel risky, using a sturdy chair or a wall for support can make a world of difference. Similarly, if full squats are tough on your knees, try half-squats or seated leg exercises that can still strengthen your lower body without the strain. Reducing the range of motion in exercises helps manage exertion levels, keeping activities safe but still beneficial. It's about working smarter, not harder, to achieve your balance goals.

Engaging with professionals for tailored advice is another key element of adapting your exercises as you age. Physical therapists and exercise specialists are like navigators in the journey of your physical health. They can assess your current balance abilities and suggest exercises that precisely fit your needs. Regular consultations ensure that your exercise regimen updates along with your physical status. These experts can offer insights into new research or techniques and introduce you to exercises that you might not have considered before. Their guidance can be particularly useful when you're dealing with new health challenges or recovering from surgery.

Lastly, embracing gentler forms of exercise can be highly beneficial. Activities like water aerobics or chair yoga provide excellent low-impact alternatives to traditional exercises. Water aerobics, for example, is a fantastic way to build strength and endurance without stressing the joints, thanks to the buoyancy of water-reducing impact. Chair yoga allows you to enjoy the flexibility and balance benefits of yoga with added support, making it accessible no matter your mobility level. These forms of exercise not only maintain physical health but also cater to it gently, respecting the body's changing needs.

By reassessing your capabilities, modifying techniques, consulting with professionals, and embracing gentler exercises, you ensure that your balance training evolves with you, supporting your well-being every step of the way. This adaptive approach allows you to continue enjoying an active, fulfilling life, filled with the activities you love, performed in a way that respects your body's needs. Keep moving, keep adjusting, and keep thriving—your balance exercises are a dynamic part of your vibrant life, changing just as you do.

10.3 Future Trends in Balance Training and Senior Health

As we glance toward the horizon, the future of balance training and overall senior health looks bright and brimming with innovation. Advances in technology are redefining what's possible, making exercises not only more effective but also more engaging. Imagine strapping on a virtual reality headset and walking through a serene forest, all from the safety of your living room. Virtual reality technology is on the cusp of revolutionising balance training by simulating real-world environments that challenge your balance without any risk of falling. This immersive experience can significantly enhance your ability to navigate everyday situations by refining your reactions and balance in a controlled, yet lifelike setting.

Moreover, advanced motion sensors are now being integrated into everyday items like shoes and walking sticks, providing real-time feedback on your posture and gait. These gadgets are designed to alert you if your balance is off, potentially preventing falls before they happen. The data collected can also be used to customise your balance training routines, focusing on specific areas where you need improvement. This tailored approach ensures that you're not just practising balance, but you're doing so in a way that directly benefits your personal mobility needs.

Turning our attention to the latest research, we're seeing exciting developments that deepen our understanding of how lifestyle factors influence balance as we age. Studies are now looking beyond simple physical exercises, exploring how diet, mental activities, and even social interactions play a role in maintaining balance. For instance, researchers are examining how omega-3 fatty acids in fish might help improve neuroplasticity, or how engaging in social activities can enhance cognitive function and, by extension, physical stability. This holistic approach to research provides a more comprehensive view of balance, emphasising that it's not just about physical strength but also overall well-being.

The development of innovative exercise equipment specifically designed for seniors is also noteworthy. These new tools are created with the understanding that safety and ease of use are paramount. Lightweight, easy-to-handle resistance bands that help build muscle strength without straining joints, and balance boards with adjustable settings to gradually increase difficulty levels, are just a couple of examples. These innovations make balance training not only safer but also more accessible, allowing more seniors to engage in these vital exercises without fear of injury.

Community and policy developments are equally important in supporting seniors in maintaining balance and mobility. Cities are beginning to recognise the need for more age-friendly public spaces, and as a result, we're seeing an increase in the number of walking paths with smooth surfaces and plenty of benches for resting. Additionally, policies are being adapted to increase access to fitness programs that include balance training as a core component. These community and legislative changes are crucial because they not only provide the resources needed for maintaining balance but also create a supportive environment that encourages an active, engaged lifestyle.

As we move forward, these trends in technology, research, equipment, and community support are setting the stage for a new era in balance training and senior health. They promise not only to enhance the effectiveness of balance exercises but also to make them a more integrated and enjoyable part of your daily life. This is about embracing innovation that not only keeps you on your feet but also enriches your life in countless ways.

As we wrap up this exploration of future trends, remember that each new development offers a stepping stone towards a lifestyle that's not just about maintaining balance but thriving. From virtual forests to smart shoes, the journey towards enhanced mobility and independence continues to evolve, promising a future where age is but a number, not a limitation. Stay tuned as we continue to navigate this exciting terrain together in the next chapter.

21-DAY BALANCE EXERCISE PROGRAM

I SN'T IT WONDERFUL HOW a few simple changes can transform your everyday life? Just like a garden that flourishes with a bit of care and attention, your balance and stability can blossom with the right exercises. That's precisely what we're going to cultivate in our 21-Day Balance Exercise Program. This program is your garden path to stronger stability, enhanced flexibility, and improved strength. It's designed with you in mind—simple enough to follow but effective enough to make a noticeable difference in how you move and feel each day.

Creating a 21-Day Balance Exercises Program for Seniors involves a combination of exercises to improve stability, strength, and flexibility. Here's a structured program that incorporates various balance exercises suitable for seniors:

Think of this program as your personal training session, where each exercise is a step towards regaining your confidence and independence. The beauty of this program lies in its simplicity and adaptability. Whether you're just starting out or you're looking to enhance your current routine, these exercises are tailored to meet you where you are. They require minimal equipment—a chair, some space, and perhaps a couple of household items like a towel or a cushion.

Getting Started with the Right Mindset

Before we jump into the exercises, let's set the stage for success. Remember, the goal here isn't perfection; it's progress. Each day that you engage in the program, you're planting seeds of improvement that will grow over time. It's important to approach this program with patience and consistency. Imagine each exercise as a building block, where day by day, you're constructing a stronger, more stable version of yourself.

The Exercises

Your 21-day journey is divided into manageable chunks, each focusing on different aspects of balance and mobility. From simple seated exercises to more dynamic standing routines, the program gradually builds in complexity and intensity. This progression is designed to gently challenge your body, enhancing your balance without overwhelming you.

The first few days focus on getting you accustomed to basic balance movements. These include simple seated leg lifts, which help strengthen your lower body and core, and arm raises to improve your upper body strength. As you grow more comfortable, you'll transition into standing exercises using a chair for support. These movements, such as standing heel raises or single-leg stands, are fantastic for engaging the larger muscle groups that play a crucial role in your balance.

As the days progress, you'll incorporate more dynamic exercises that mimic daily activities. For example, walking heel-to-toe, which can significantly improve your gait and stability, especially when navigating uneven surfaces like a grassy backyard or a bumpy sidewalk. To keep things interesting and challenging, you'll also try some balance exercises on different surfaces. This variety not only keeps your routine fresh but also trains your body to adapt to various environments, enhancing your overall mobility.

Interactive Element: Reflective Journaling

Keeping a Balance Diary

To maximise the benefits of this program, I encourage you to keep a balance diary. This isn't just about tracking which exercises you've done; it's about noting how you felt doing them, any improvements you've noticed, or particular challenges you faced. This reflective practice can be incredibly rewarding. It allows you to see your progress over the days, which can be a huge motivational boost. It also helps you understand your body better, making you more attuned to how different exercises affect your balance and stability.

This 21-day program is more than just about preventing falls—it's about empowering you to lead a more active, independent life. By dedicating just a few minutes each day to these exercises, you're not only enhancing your physical health but also boosting your confidence and well-being. So, let's step forward with enthusiasm and a positive spirit, ready to embrace each day's activities with the knowledge that you're doing something wonderful for yourself.

Tips for Safety and Effectiveness

Embarking on a new exercise regimen, especially one focused on improving balance, can feel like a refreshing start to enhancing your overall health and independence. As you move through the 21-day program, keeping some key safety and effectiveness tips in mind will ensure that you not only benefit fully from the exercises but also enjoy them without any hitches. Let's talk about some smart strategies to keep you on track and injury-free.

One of the simplest yet most effective ways to ensure safety during your balance exercises is using a chair for support. In the early stages of the program, or whenever trying a new exercise that feels challenging, having a sturdy chair by your side offers a reliable safety net. You can use it to steady yourself as you perform standing exercises or even perform some exercises while seated until you feel confident enough to do them standing. This isn't just about preventing falls; it's about giving you the confidence to perform exercises with proper form, which is crucial for them to be effective. So, think of that chair as your trusty exercise buddy—always there to support you, no matter what.

Now, let's talk about what's on your feet. Wearing proper footwear cannot be overstated when it comes to balance exercises. A good pair of supportive shoes provides a stable base that can make a significant difference in your ability to maintain balance. Look for shoes with non-slip soles that offer good ankle support. They should fit well—not too tight, not too loose—and provide adequate cushioning to absorb impacts, which will reduce stress on your joints. This kind of footwear not only enhances your performance but also protects you from potential injuries, making your balance practice both safe and enjoyable.

Progression is another cornerstone of a successful exercise program. It's important to increase the duration and difficulty of your exercises gradually. As you become more comfortable with the initial exercises, start challenging yourself a bit more each day, but always within your comfort zone. This might mean holding a pose for a few seconds longer, adding more repetitions, or trying a slightly more complex movement. Incremental increases will help improve your strength and balance steadily, reducing the risk of injuries that can come from doing too much too soon. Remember, the goal is steady progress, not instant perfection.

Hydration is often overlooked in exercise routines, but it plays a pivotal role, especially for seniors. Ensuring you drink enough water before and after your exercises helps keep your muscles and joints lubricated, aids in recovery, and keeps your body functioning optimally. Dehydration can lead to tiredness, dizziness, and muscle cramps, all of which can be detrimental when you're trying to maintain or improve balance. So, keep a bottle of water handy during your workouts, and sip regularly.

Lastly, always listen to your body. This is perhaps the most personalised piece of advice because only you know exactly how you feel during an exercise. If you experience pain or discomfort, stop what you're doing and assess. Pain is your body's way of signaling that something isn't right, and ignoring it can lead to more serious injuries. If a particular exercise consistently causes discomfort, consider modifying it or consulting with a healthcare provider for an alternative. Your exercise routine should challenge you, yes, but it should not cause pain.

By integrating these tips into your daily exercise routine, you create a safe and effective environment for improving your balance and strength. These strategies not only help in preventing injuries but also make the exercises more enjoyable and beneficial. Remember, the goal of this program is to enhance your independence and quality of life through improved balance and stability. Each day, with each exercise, you are taking active steps toward that goal, building a stronger, more confident you.

Week 1: Introduction to Balance (5 minutes/day)

Day 1-2:

1. **Heel-to-Toe Walk** – 1 minute

2. **Single-Leg Stand (with support)** – 1 minute (30 seconds each leg)

3. **Chair-Assisted Marching** – 2 minutes

4. **Standing Side Leg Lift (with support)** – 1 minute (30 seconds each leg)

Day 3:

- Rest Day

Day 4-5:

1. **Heel-to-Toe Walk** – 1 minute

2. **Single-Leg Stand (with support)** – 1 minute (30 seconds each leg)

3. **Chair-Assisted Marching** – 2 minutes

4. **Standing Side Leg Lift (with support)** – 1 minute (30 seconds each leg)

Day 6:

1. **Heel-to-Toe Walk** – 1 minute

2. **Single-Leg Stand (with support)** – 1 minute (30 seconds each leg)

3. **Chair-Assisted Marching** – 2 minutes

4. **Standing Side Leg Lift (with support)** – 1 minute (30 seconds each leg)

Day 7:

- Rest Day

Week 2: Building Confidence (7 minutes/day)

Day 8-9:

1. **Heel-to-Toe Walk** – 1 minute

2. **Single-Leg Stand (with or without support)** – 2 minutes (1 minute each leg)

3. **Chair-Assisted Marching** – 2 minutes

4. **Standing Side Leg Lift (with support)** – 1 minute (30 seconds each leg)

5. **Heel Raises (with support)** – 1 minute

Day 10:

- Rest Day

Day 11-12:

1. **Heel-to-Toe Walk** – 1 minute

2. **Single-Leg Stand (with or without support)** – 2 minutes (1 minute each leg)

3. **Chair-Assisted Marching** – 2 minutes

4. **Standing Side Leg Lift (with support)** – 1 minute (30 seconds each leg)

5. **Heel Raises (with support)** – 1 minute

Day 13:

1. **Heel-to-Toe Walk** – 1 minute

2. **Single-Leg Stand (with or without support)** – 2 minutes (1 minute each leg)

3. **Chair-Assisted Marching** – 2 minutes

4. **Standing Side Leg Lift (with support)** – 1 minute (30 seconds each leg)

5. **Heel Raises (with support)** – 1 minute

Day 14:

- Rest Day

Week 3: Building Endurance (10 minutes/day)

Day 15-16:

1. **Heel-to-Toe Walk** – 2 minutes

2. **Single-Leg Stand (with or without support)** – 2 minutes (1 minute each leg)

3. **Chair-Assisted Marching** – 2 minutes

4. **Standing Side Leg Lift (with support)** – 1 minute (30 seconds each leg)

5. **Heel Raises (with support)** – 2 minutes

6. **Seated Knee Lifts** – 1 minute

Day 17:

- Rest Day

Day 18-19:

1. **Heel-to-Toe Walk** – 2 minutes

2. **Single-Leg Stand (with or without support)** – 2 minutes (1 minute each leg)

3. **Chair-Assisted Marching** – 2 minutes

4. **Standing Side Leg Lift (with support)** – 1 minute (30 seconds each leg)

5. **Heel Raises (with support)** – 2 minutes

6. **Seated Knee Lifts** – 1 minute

Day 20:

1. **Heel-to-Toe Walk** – 2 minutes

2. **Single-Leg Stand (with or without support)** – 2 minutes (1 minute each leg)

3. **Chair-Assisted Marching** – 2 minutes

4. **Standing Side Leg Lift (with support)** – 1 minute (30 seconds each leg)

5. **Heel Raises (with support)** – 2 minutes

6. **Seated Knee Lifts** – 1 minute

Day 21:

- Rest Day

Exercise Descriptions

1. **Heel-to-Toe Walk:** Walk in a straight line, placing the heel of one foot directly in front of the toes of the other foot. Use a wall or chair for balance if needed.

2. **Single-Leg Stand (with support):** Stand on one leg while holding onto a chair for support. Aim to hold for 30 seconds, then switch legs. As you progress, try to balance without support.

3. **Chair-Assisted Marching:** While seated or standing, march in place, lifting your knees as high as comfortably possible.

4. **Standing Side Leg Lift (with support):** Stand with one hand on a chair for balance, lift one leg out to the side, lower it, and repeat. Switch sides.

5. **Heel Raises (with support):** Stand behind a chair, hold the back for support, and rise up onto your toes. Lower back down and repeat.

6. **Seated Knee Lifts:** While seated in a chair, lift one knee towards your chest, lower it, and repeat with the other leg.

Congratulations on reaching the end of your 21-day Balance Exercises journey! Your dedication and perseverance have paid off, and you've successfully embraced a routine that promotes balance, stability, and overall well-being.

As we conclude this chapter, these tips form the pillars that support your journey through the 21-Day Balance Exercise Program. They ensure that as you progress, you do so with care, making each step forward as safe and effective as possible.

CONCLUSION

WELL, MY FRIEND, HERE we are at the end of our journey together through the pages of this book. It's been quite the adventure, hasn't it? We've covered a lot of ground, from the very basics of balance exercises to more advanced techniques, and everything in between. I hope you've found each chapter not just informative but also inspiring as you've taken steps to enhance your stability and regain your independence.

Reflecting back on our discussions, we've learned how crucial balance is, not just for preventing falls, but for living a full and active life. We've explored how the body's balance system works and how it changes as we age. More importantly, we've discovered that with regular practice and the right exercises, you can significantly improve your balance.

Remember, the essence of this book isn't just about avoiding falls—it's about empowering you to lead a life that's as vibrant and fulfilling as possible. It's about making those golden years truly shine. Every exercise, every tip, and every piece of advice has been geared towards helping you feel more confident and secure on your feet.

I know that starting something new, especially something like a balance exercise routine can sometimes feel a bit daunting. But I hope that with the step-by-step guides and the personal insights shared, you feel like you have a companion in me.

Always remember, you're not alone on this path. Just like any good journey, it's always more enjoyable and meaningful when shared.

As we wrap things up, I urge you to keep the momentum going. Use what you've learned here to keep challenging yourself every day, even in small ways. Whether it's trying out a new exercise or simply incorporating more movement into your daily routine, every little bit counts. And if you ever feel like you're slipping or need a refresher, just flip back through these pages. This book is here to be your guide and reminder that you have the power to maintain and even improve your balance.

Thank you for trusting me to be a part of your journey to a more stable and confident life. Keep stepping forward with courage and cheer, knowing that each step you take is a testament to your strength and resilience. Here's to many more years of enjoying the balance you've worked so hard to achieve!

Keep moving, keep balancing, and most importantly, keep enjoying every step of this wonderful journey. You've got this!

MAKE A DIFFERENCE WITH YOUR REVIEW

If you found this book helpful, informative, or useful, then please do leave a review on Google or Amazon, as it helps get this book out to more people who can also benefit just as you did.

Make a Difference with Your Review

Now you have everything you need to find relief, balance, and independence, it's time to pass on your newfound knowledge and show other readers where they can find the same help.

Simply by leaving your honest opinion of this book on Amazon, you'll show other seniors where they can find the information they're looking for and pass their passion for Balance Exercises moving forward.

Thank you for your help. The practice of Balance Exercises for Seniors is kept alive when we pass on our knowledge – and you're helping me to do just that.

Your review can make a difference for someone who's on the fence about starting their journey into Balance Exercises. Share your thoughts and let them know how this book has impacted your life.

Remember, your experiences and insights can be the guiding light for others seeking the benefits of Balance Exercises.

Thank you once again for being a part of this journey and for sharing the love of Balance Exercises with others.

Your biggest fan, Laurel Harris

Scan the QR code to leave your review!

OTHER BOOKS IN THE SERIES

Thank you so much for joining me on this journey through Balance Exercises for Seniors.

If you are interested in any other books in the Fitness and Self Help for Seniors Series, please check out my other books below – thank you.

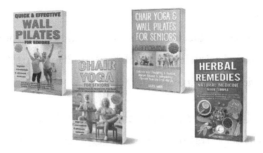

REFERENCES

- Crescent Fields Senior Living. (n.d.). Why should senior citizens perform balance exercises? Crescent Fields Senior Living. https://crescentfieldsseniorliving.com/why-should-senior-citizens-perform-balance-exercises/

- National Institute on Aging. (n.d.). Older adults and balance problems. National Institute on Aging. https://www.nia.nih.gov/health/falls-and-falls-prevention/older-adults-and-balance-problems

- Medical News Today. (n.d.). Neuroplasticity exercises: 5 tips to try. Medical News Today. https://www.medicalnewstoday.com/articles/neuroplasticity-exercises#:~:text=Activities%20such%20as%20making%20music,cognitive%20decline%20in%20older%20age

- National Center for Biotechnology Information. (2015). Taking balance training for older adults one step further. https://www.ncbi.nlm.nih.gov/pmc/articles/PMC4419050/

- Healthline. (n.d.). Exercise plan for seniors: Strength, stretching, and balance. Healthline. https://www.healthline.com/health/everyday-fitness/senior-workouts

- Wellness NIFS. (n.d.). Top 5 balance training tools for seniors. https://wellness.nifs.org/blog/top-5-balance-training-tools-for-seniors

- Johns Hopkins Arthritis Center. (n.d.). Role of exercise in arthritis management. https://www.hopkinsarthritis.org/patient-corner/disease-management/role-of-exercise-in-arthritis-management/

- SilverSneakers. (n.d.). 5 warm-up exercises for seniors: Tips from the experts. SilverSneakers. https://www.silversneakers.com/blog/warm-up-exercise/

- National Center for Biotechnology Information. (2022). Effectiveness of Tai Chi for health promotion of older adults. https://www.ncbi.nlm.nih.gov/pmc/articles/PMC9644143/

- Johns Hopkins Medicine. (n.d.). Fall prevention: Balance and strength exercises for older adults. https://www.hopkinsmedicine.org/health/wellness-and-prevention/fall-prevention-exercises

- Caregiver Solutions. (n.d.). Eight chair exercises for older adults with limited mobility. https://caregiversolutions.ca/health-and-wellness/eight-chair-exercises-for-older-adults-with-limited-mobility/

- National Center for Biotechnology Information. (2015). Taking balance training for older adults one step further. https://www.ncbi.nlm.nih.gov/pmc/articles/PMC4419050/

- Harvard Health. (n.d.). The best core exercises for older adults. Harvard Health Publishing. https://www.health.harvard.edu/staying-healthy/the-best-core-exercises-for-older-adults

- National Center for Biotechnology Information. (2022). Acute and chronic effects of supervised flexibility training.

https://www.ncbi.nlm.nih.gov/pmc/articles/PMC9779245/

- SilverSneakers. (n.d.). 8 yoga poses to improve balance and stability. SilverSneakers. https://www.silversneakers.com/blog/yoga-seniors-poses-improve-balance/

- National Center for Biotechnology Information. (2019). Pilates versus resistance training on trunk strength and balance adaptations in older women: A randomized controlled trial. https://www.ncbi.nlm.nih.gov/pmc/articles/PMC6859004/

- National Center for Biotechnology Information. (2022). Effectiveness of Tai Chi for health promotion of older adults. https://www.ncbi.nlm.nih.gov/pmc/articles/PMC9644143/

- Means, K. M. (1996). The obstacle course. Journal of Rehabilitation Research and Development, 33(4), 371-380. https://www.rehab.research.va.gov/jour/96/33/4/pdf/means.pdf

- PubMed. (2019). Does integrated cognitive and balance (dual-task) training improve balance in older adults? https://pubmed.ncbi.nlm.nih.gov/31010491/

- University of Mississippi Medical Center. (n. d.). Vestibular (balance) exercises. University of Mississippi. https://www.umc.edu/Healthcare/ENT/Patient-Handouts/Adult/Otology/Vestibular_Exercises.html

- National Center for Biotechnology Information. (2015). Taking balance training for older adults one step further. https://www.ncbi.nlm.nih.gov/pmc/articles/PMC4419050/

- National Center for Biotechnology Information. (2016). Mindfulness-based interventions for older adults. https://www.ncbi.nlm.nih.gov/pmc/articles/PMC4868399/

- WebMD. (n.d.). Safe outdoor exercises for older adults. WebMD. https://www.webmd.com/healthy-aging/ss/slideshow-exercises-older-adults-can-safely-do-outside

- Public Safety Medical. (2017). Selecting and effectively using a stability ball. Public Safety Medical. https://publicsafetymed.com/wp-content/uploads/2017/05/Using-Stablility-balls.pdf

- Crescent Fields Senior Living. (n.d.). Why should senior citizens perform balance exercises? Crescent Fields Senior Living. https://crescentfieldsseniorliving.com/why-should-senior-citizens-perform-balance-exercises/

- Healthline. (n.d.). Exercise plan for seniors: Strength, stretching, and balance. Healthline. https://www.healthline.com/health/everyday-fitness/senior-workouts

- iAdvance Senior Care. (n.d.). How technology can support senior exercise and physical activity. iAdvance Senior Care. https://www.iadvanceseniorcare.com/how-technology-can-support-senior-exercise-and-physical-activity/

- YMCA. (n.d.). Moving for better balance exercise program. YMCA. https://www.ymca.org/what-we-do/healthy-living/fitness/older-adults/better-balance

- South Dakota State University Extension. (n.d.). Overcoming barriers to physical activity while aging. South Dakota State University Extension. https://extension.sdstate.edu/overcoming-barriers-physical-activity-while-aging

- A Place for Mom. (n.d.). 8 gentle exercises for seniors with arthritis. A Place for Mom. https://www.aplaceformom.com/caregiver-resources/articles/gentle-exercises-for-seniors-with-arthritis

- National Council on Aging. (n.d.). Evidence-based falls prevention programs. National Council on Aging. https://www.ncoa.org/article/evi-dence-based-falls-prevention-programs

- PubMed. (2018). Cognitive behavioural therapy for fear of falling and older adults. https://pubmed.ncbi.nlm.nih.gov/29471428/

- MedlinePlus. (n.d.). Nutrition for older adults. MedlinePlus. https://medlineplus.gov/nutritionforolderadults.html

- National Center for Biotechnology Information. (2023). The effects of exercise for cognitive function in older adults. https://www.ncbi.nlm.nih.gov/pmc/articles/PMC9858649/

- National Center for Biotechnology Information. (2019). The role of water homeostasis in muscle function and older adults. https://www.ncbi.nlm.nih.gov/pmc/articles/PMC6723611/

- HelpGuide. (n.d.). Relaxation techniques for stress re-lief. HelpGuide. https://www.helpguide.org/articles/stress/relax-ation-techniques-for-stress-relief.htm

- Crescent Fields Senior Living. (n.d.). Why should senior citizens perform balance exercises? Crescent Fields Senior Living. https://crescentfieldsseniorliving.com/why-should-senior-citi-zens-perform-balance-exercises/

- GaitBetter. (n.d.). The vital role of dynamic balance in promoting safe gait in older adults. GaitBetter. https://www.gaitbetter.com/dynam-ic-balance-elderly-gait-safety/

- National Institute on Aging. (n.d.). Older adults and balance problems. National Institute on Aging. https://www.nia.nih.gov/health/falls-an d-falls-prevention/older-adults-and-balance-problems

- A Place for Mom. (n.d.). 8 gentle exercises for seniors with arthri-tis. A Place for Mom. https://www.aplaceformom.com/caregiver-resources/articles/gentle-exercises-for-seniors-with-arthritis

Made in United States
Troutdale, OR
12/26/2024

27305683R00086